THE WORLD'S BEST-KEPT DIET SECRETS

LOSE WEIGHT QUICKLY, SAFELY AND PERMANENTLY

DIANE IRONS

JOHN BLAKE

Published by John Blake Publishing Ltd,
3 Bramber Court, 2 Bramber Road,
London W14 9PB, England

First published in hardback 2000

ISBN 1 903402 344

British Library Cataloguing-in-Publication Data:

A catalogue record for this book is
available from the British Library.

Typeset by t2

Printed in Great Britain by
Creative Print and Design (Wales),
Ebbw Vale, Gwent.

3 5 7 9 10 8 6 4

Papers used by John Blake Publishing Limited are natural,
recyclable products made from wood grown in sustainable forests. The manufacturing
processes conform to the environmental regulations of the country of origin.

Table of Contents

Dedication

To David and Kirk

Conversion Table

Dry Measures

1 cup is equal to 8 ounces

Liquid Measures

1 cup is equal to 8fl oz.

Acknowledgements

So many people have contributed to this book by sharing their stories, their expertise, their time, and most importantly, their hearts. My deepest appreciation goes to my many colleagues and friends, who upon hearing of my quest for concrete answers to the conundrum of dieting and weight loss, led me to the most powerful and precise resources.

I am extremely grateful to my publicist and dear friend, Renee Calomino, for her dedication and intuitive knowledge of my intentions. I consider our relationship an invaluable gift in both my life and my work.

Finally, there are not enough words in which to thank my husband, David, my life's love, and my son, Kirk, my "lucky star".

Introduction

When it comes to losing weight and keeping it off, what really works? I have been looking for the answer ever since I started modelling at the age of thirteen and had to fight my own weight problems. I looked to the most beautiful bodies in the business to give me the answers and direction. When I became a reporter and image consultant, regardless of the story I was covering, at the end of the interview, if there was a body I admired, I wanted to know how it happened. Have you always been slim? If not, how did you get the weight off? How do you stay so disciplined? What do you eat? What do you avoid? Is your family slim? How do you lose weight quickly when a film or modelling job comes up? What's your favorite low-calorie recipe? Usually, when the microphone comes down, the reserves fall away and the stars shared their secrets with me.

It was not just celebrities who intrigued me. My nationally broadcast "lifestyle" shows featured "real" people who shared with me both their triumphs and tragedies. Again, their weight played important roles in their relationships, self-esteem, and career choices. In my research for this book, I interviewed men and women who spent countless pounds on books, pills, pricey diet and exercise programmes, and other promises. I tracked down friends who had friends with important life-changing stories.

This book is a compilation of tips from famous celebrities and "real" people. I have talked to trainers to find out the best exercises and equipment for the least money. I have worked with nutritionists, physicians, and chemists to find the natural supplements that are important aids to weight loss.

I hope I have covered everything. Probably like you, I have tired of diet books that tell one story, one struggle, one philosophy. Although these books are well-intentioned, what worked for me, him or her may not drive you to your own answer. My hope is that you will draw on your own inspiration and create your own lifestyle changes from my pursuits.

In order to get the intimate stories in this book, I had to promise my subjects total anonymity, so I have identified them only by their first name, age, and the amount of weight they have lost. Weight losses ranged from just 10 pounds to almost 200 pounds, but the weight must have stayed off at least five years to be included. Like many of us, my contacts had often lost and regained weight several times before finally reaching their permanent goals.

Use this book to find the keys to success that exist within the framework of your own personality. These are the tools and information you will need to get there, but it is you who will do the work and reap the fabulous rewards to come.

Chapter One

Getting Started

So What's the Secret?

Diets Are Like Spokes on a Wheel

When we hear about someone who's lost weight and kept it off, we all want to know how they did it. What was the secret to their success? I have spent years attempting to unlock these secrets in my work as an image researcher and journalist. From my "other" life in modelling, I have been witness to great successes of permanent weight loss as well as seeing highly lucrative careers ruined by food obsessions.

Let me set you straight before we get started. I did not find one diet that is going to work for everyone. I have interviewed hundreds of individuals who have successfully lost weight and kept it off. They did it by charting their own course. Most diet books are one person's experience or opinion, and at the very least anecdotal. This storytelling of "what worked for me" has sold a lot of books. Physicians also put forth dieting advice which is theory-based, and did not work for the majority of the successful dieters I interviewed. These diets failed because they were too complicated to follow, too prohibitive, or too expensive. Sometimes they worked for the short term, but could not sustain long-term results. These doctors are not gods or gurus, and my interviews conclude that diets are more about lifestyle change than simply a matter of science and chemistry. Diets are about life.

What's Your Story?

It comes as no surprise that each dieter has a different philosophy of "ideal" weight. Rather than following weight charts, successful dieters chose to rely on criteria such as the weight at which they felt their most comfortable, pre-pregnancy weights, etc. Their stories included cruelty, abandonment, embarrassment, and discrimination.

Playing Mind Games

When I asked people their initial feelings before embarking on a diet programme, the overwhelming response was "anxiety", a reply echoed by both successful and failed dieters. Dieters feel enormous trepidation and a fear of being overwhelmed. It hits them hardest when they start out, no matter what their size, goal, or planned regime.

"I was afraid that my obsession with chocolate would not allow me to get to my final goal. It was only recognising that I could have one piece of chocolate a day that let me get through it."

Mary, age 38, 25 pounds lost

"My fears were due to my extreme hate of exercise. I knew that exercise was necessary for weight loss, but for me it was just too overwhelming to think about getting geared up for a diet and exercise programme at the same time. My solution was to not join a gym, but start walking whenever I could. I got hooked on it, and now I run three miles a day and love how it makes me feel."

Frank, age 45, 53 pounds lost

Take Charge

You need to come to the decision that food has dictated how you live your life for far too long. It probably has coloured every component of your daily activity. Those who have found their weight loss to be successful permanently talk about a feeling of power, where previously there was only powerlessness.

Wipe the Slate Clean

Successful weight loss begins with the end of doubts, regrets, and remorse — no more of "what if?" "why did I?" and "if only." It really doesn't matter what you did yesterday or ten years ago. It doesn't matter how old you are or how many pounds you want to lose. To accomplish your goal, it is important for you to set your site on mini goals. Losing eighty pounds is tremendously scary, and yet making yourself ten pounds lighter is not only attainable, but a goal you can live with for now.

Pace Yourself

Eat what you want, and eat it when you want. The reason why diet programmes have such a high failure rate is partly due to their regimentation. Taking away your favourite foods only makes you feel even more deprived. You won't go too long before those cravings for pizza and chocolate overcome your every waking minute. Look, even if you hate brussel sprouts, any diet that said you could never have them again would make you think about them all the time. Next thing you know, you'll be craving them. You'll be hitting the grocery stores looking for brussel sprouts!

There is no "bad" food, and although some foods are better than others, there are no "good" foods. Get those words out of your vocabulary, and keep them out. Everyone has their own rhythm that feels right to them. Also, only you know when you're truly hungry. Eating by the clock is just not workable for most successful dieters.

3

Start a Food Diary

The only way you'll win this battle is to figure out what triggers your overeating. Even if you head into a binge, putting your feelings down on paper will create a commonality that will help you understand the nature of your weight problems. Calories have a way of creeping up. Research done by the American Dietetic Association found that dieters who were not successful after countless weight loss efforts were underestimating their calories by as much as 300 per cent. They also thought they exercised much more than they really did. If it's too hard to keep a daily journal, at least try to keep track of two weekdays and one weekend day. Note such things as mood, fat and calorie content of what you eat, what you were doing or feeling before you ate, and how you felt afterwards (satisfied, sad, mad, etc.).

Know Your Body Fat

Your weight is important, but the amount of fat in your body is equally important. Combining both gives a more accurate picture of overall body fitness. If you have an acceptable weight but too much body fat, your health could be in jeopardy. The USDA recommendation is that no more than 30 per cent of your daily caloric intake come from fat.

Here's how to measure:
1. Using a millimetre ruler, pinch the fold of skin directly in front of your armpit, vertically in at the front of your thigh, and vertically an inch to the side of your belly button. Hold the ruler away from your body, as straight as possible.

2. Add all three measurements together.

3. Your total should be no higher than 100. Higher than that means that you have more than 30 percent body fat.

Do You Know Your BMI?

The body mass index (BMI) measures the relationship between your weight and your height. Here's how you find yours:

1. Multiply your weight in pounds by .45 to get kilos.

2. Take your height in inches and multiply by 0.0254 to get metres.

3. Multiply that number by itself.

4. Divide this into your weight in kilos. This is your BMI. The accepted healthy range is from 19 to 25 according to the National Examination Survey.

How Much Should You Weigh?

Forget the complicated chart! An easy way to figure out what you should weigh is to allow 100 pounds for the first five feet of height and five pounds for each additional inch. Most charts calculate that ten pounds below that is just about right for small frames, and ten pounds above is normal for larger frames. But don't get married to that. You know where you feel your healthiest.

There are lots of other criteria to consider also. Yours might be getting back into your wedding or ball dress. With most people I've interviewed, they usually cite their high school weight as their ideal. From what I've observed, it's been self-sabotaging to get stuck at a certain weight. However, adhering to a weight range seems to work for most successful dieters no matter how much they've lost. For some it's ten pounds and for others it's just five. I remember interviewing the late Ava Gabor who weighed herself twice a day. If she weighed one more pound than the previous day's weight she cut out all bread and dessert that day. She told me that she just couldn't trust herself otherwise. That's pretty stringent, but is pretty typical of anyone I've ever interviewed whose career was based on their looks.

Don't Get Too Technical

The problem with most diet books and diet programmes is that they are so complicated and difficult to follow that the dieters I interviewed found themselves constantly having to think about what they ate. This result proved a negative for the majority of them. They were literally consumed with thoughts of food, which caused them to overeat.

"I've been on more 'stylised' diets than I want to count. Trying to figure out what to eat next made me crazy! I had food on the mind all the time. Only when I could finally sit down to a meal and eat what appealed to me at that very moment did I feel like a 'real' person."

Tasha, age 48, 60 pounds lost

Tasha is typical of successful dieters who told me that choosing foods that felt "right" at the time, were convenient, etc., were what they needed. Some even labelled it "self-permission". These dieters were more successful when they discovered the tools they needed for their weight loss. They regarded the more complex diet programmes as complicated architectural blueprints that made no sense to their lives or lifestyles.

> **Whenever I got angry** I would eat and eat until the feelings went away. My head would tell me not to do it. On an intellectual level, I knew what was happening, but I was powerless to the quick fix.
>
> **Peter, age 64, 110 pounds lost**

Listen to Your Body

Your body will signal you with what is wrong and what it needs. Sometimes it will scream at you for help. For example, women report craving certain foods (usually chocolate) about a week before their menstrual cycles. Research indicates that this is due to a deficiency of magnesium. In another person, fatigue may mean that more protein is needed in their diet. Also, craving "comfort" foods like bread, pastry, or crackers could simply indicate boredom or stress.

"I can't tell you the number of days I would come home from a particularly bad day at work, and head directly to that bag of chips or crackers. More times than I care to admit, it would be before taking my coat off or greeting my family. Learning to meditate for ten minutes after work helped me to avoid an entire night of bingeing."

Sid, age 39, 82 pounds lost

"Realising that taking two aspirin alleviated my headaches more efficiently (and with a lot less calories) than a pint of ice cream or an entire cheesecake allowed me to take charge of my health and my weight."

Marsha, age 52, 36 pounds lost

Develop a Reward System

Successful dieters have found that having something to look forward to at the end of each milestone (first five pounds, getting through a tough weekend, etc.) helped to mentally and emotionally shorten the cycles of long-term success.

"I realised that I had to look at myself in an entirely different way. Somehow over the years I had put myself on the shelf and didn't feel I was worthy enough, partly because of my weight, to treat

7

myself to the 'little luxuries'. So even though I had a tremendous amount of weight to lose, I began to act like those high-maintenance babes I had so long been envious of. For every five pounds I lost, I had my nails done (even pedicures), had my hair highlighted, and made inexpensive 'bauble' purchases. They made me feel good about myself, which were feelings that I had long ago forgotten. Looking forward to those little rewards helped me to stay on track during the toughest days."

Marge, age 44, 77 pounds lost

Accept the Consequences

Just as important as rewarding themselves through the milestones of their diet, it was equally beneficial for dieters to accept some form of retribution for slipping. For some it was as simple as not allowing themselves their daily treat for two or three days, while for others it was more punitive.

"I had to take 'just this once' completely out of my vocabulary. When I went off my diet I would literally punish myself. I would climb five floors to my job, make my own coffee rather than buying it, etc. I had to feel that there was going to be more of a cause and effect than just gaining back the weight. I usually incorporated something that would make up for my 'slip up'. It worked for me."

Alan, age 27, 48 pounds lost

It's a Gift You Give Yourself

Think of your weight-loss programme as the most important gift you have ever given yourself. Only when you take away the "poor me routine" can you really just grow up and get on with it. Now is the time to experience new tastes. Enjoy the entire experience of eating, and get the most from every morsel. This will eliminate feelings of deprivation.

Talk Back to Your Head

When something goes wrong in our lives, those voices in our head start in. They try to tell us that the only way we'll get over that disappointment or loneliness is with the antidote of food. Tell yourself that you've had these feelings before, and you've lived through it. No amount of food will take away these feelings. In fact, it will only make you feel worse afterwards. Then start talking yourself into a better body.

Gender Differences

"Women tend to binge when they are angry or sad, or they use food as a source of comfort when alone or depressed. Obese men were found to binge in positive social situations when celebrating or encouraged by others to eat."

— *Elle* **magazine**

Create a Contract

Take the time to write out a contract with yourself. These 10 rules are a good start for terms you can live up to. Add your own resolutions to this list if you'd like. Take it out whenever you are tempted to break the terms of the contract.

1. I resolve to eat only when I am truly hungry.

2. I resolve to try a new fruit or vegetable.

3. I resolve to treat myself to a forbidden food once a week.

4. I resolve to limit consumption of diet beverages and other chemicals.

5. I resolve to drink 8 to 10 glasses of water daily.

6. I resolve to exercise at least 3 times a week.

7. I resolve to replace a red meat meal with tofu.

8. I resolve to accept responsibility for my actions.

9. I resolve to think before I eat.

10. I resolve to take it one day at a time.

My name:_____

My current weight:_____

My goal weight:_____

Reason for losing weight:_____

Signed:_____

Date:_____

Understand Why You Overeat

Everyone knows that food is a great tranquilliser. It creates a buffer zone from the hurts and issues that plague everyone's life experiences. Understanding why they turn to food rather than solving the problems has worked for the chronic binge eaters I interviewed.

"My weight gain came when my last child left for college. I was left with an emptiness that I filled with food. The foods that I chose were the typical comfort foods like cakes, biscuits, and the creamiest pastries I could find. Fifty pounds later I finally came to terms with it, and replaced the 'empty foods' with my 'empty nest' realisation."

Bunny, age 56, 50 pounds lost

"When I married my husband I weighed 115 pounds. At 5'4" I wore a size twelve and thought that I had a pretty good body. My husband never complimented me, but continually put me up against other women. This affected my esteem in such a way that I started to eat as a way of getting back at him. The more he criticised, the more I ate. When he finally left me I weighed in at 188 pounds. When I realised that I could never base my appearance on other's expectations, and that I was good 'as is', I was able to take control of my weight and my life."

Portia, age 36, 62 pounds lost

Stop Fighting Nature

When setting your goal weight, try not to squeeze into some "ideal" mould that you've seen in the movies or a fashion magazine. If you've never been a size eight, chances are you are not meant to be that small.

Be Aware of Seasonal Challenges

A lot of us gain weight during the colder months. The average gain is between 5 and 7 pounds, usually gained around the holidays. The type of foods we eat also make a major contribution to this weight gain. We are less likely to reach for that salad when we're chilly. The dieters I interviewed told me that their biggest diet challenges came during the winter months. Outside activities are usually curtailed, and exercise programmes drop off.

"I couldn't get my body warm enough. I guess I tried to compensate for this by reaching for heavy foods. When I tried to warm myself up with coffee, it just made me jittery, and again, I would use food to calm me down. Now that I've lost the weight, I keep bouillon cubes on hand, and sip broth throughout the day. At just six calories a cup, I keep myself warm and satisfied all day long."

Paul, age 47, 23 pounds lost

"I hate the whole gym scene, but I couldn't get myself out the door in the freezing temperatures and on icy roads to walk the hour I do in nice weather. Investing in a treadmill and keeping it in sight was a lifesaver in keeping my weight off."

Moe, age 33, 18 pounds lost

Check That Stress Level

Almost everyone, no matter what their lifestyle, no matter how much money in the bank, told me that one of the greatest challenges to their weight loss was coping with stress. Whether it was a client's demands, the kids fighting, or even trying to balance the cheque book, a quick trip to the kitchen was the only way they could diffuse the tension building up inside. So we eat, and get even more stressed out.

The weight loss industry makes profits of over $40 billion a year!

Change Your Relationship with Food

Dieters who maintain long-term weight loss have had to come to terms with the role that food plays in their daily lives. Only when they were able to put food back into its proper place were they able to not only lose the excess pounds, but also resume a normal lifestyle.

"The whole issue of food was taking up too much of my time. There were more days than I care to count when I would wake up thinking of food, praying to God to keep me away from the fridge. I was unable to work, to think, even to move. Previously, I had been able to quit smoking and overcome a prescription drug dependency. This was harder because obviously I couldn't eliminate food from my life."

Chuck, age 26, 120 pounds lost

Expect a Rocky Road

The final success is the acceptance that there is bound to be failure along the way to reaching your goal. Eliminating that "all or nothing" attitude and planning for those inevitable glitches will allow you to look at the long-range plan you've made. When you do break your diet, you're able to pick yourself up, dust yourself off, and get going again.

"When I would eat one biscuit, I would figure that I had blown the whole day, so instead of eating just that one biscuit, I would devour the entire box. Now I allow myself to have one, even two biscuits, and not feel that I've taken a big setback. Allowing myself to enjoy the occasional treat keeps me from feeling alienated from society."

Pat, age 34, 40 pounds lost

Never Skip Meals

Skipping any meal sets you up to overeat at the next meal. With that said, though, many dieters did not adhere to three meals a day. Some ate just twice a day while others chose to eat six mini-meals throughout the day. The key is to eat at regular intervals.

"I have a problem of going in and out of the refrigerator and the kitchen cabinets all day long. What worked for me was taking the models from *Sports Illustrated*, cutting off their heads, and sticking my head on top of their bodies. I stuck a picture on each of my 'dangerous' cabinets as well as on the refrigerator."

Sandy, age 30, 25 pounds lost

Don't Call It a Diet

People who have lost weight and kept off the weight they lost have done so by pretty much sticking to whatever tools they used to take the weight off in the first place. Even after reaching their goals, successful dieters continued to watch the fat content of the foods they ate, measured portions, and maintained an exercise programme.

"As soon as I started going back to my old style of eating, the weight started climbing again. What keeps my weight at bay is using the programme I used to lose the weight during the week, and enjoying some extras on the weekend. Yeah, come Monday I may be a couple of pounds up, but I know that it will come off by getting right back on track. It gives me something to look forward to. I'd go crazy if I didn't have my Saturday night dinners out."

Mac, age 35, 58 pounds lost

Think Thin

Using visualisation seems to work in getting many dieters over the humps of a long-term diet. Here's how it works: picture yourself at the weight you'd like to be, dressed in the clothes you've always wanted to wear, doing the things you've always wanted to do. Now picture how others will react to you at your new weight. Concentrate on the feelings these thoughts evoke.

Set the Scene for Success

Always eat in a calm atmosphere. Thriller movies, loud and fast music, and crowded places cause us to eat faster than we should. They also make us less aware of what we're eating. Always sit down when eating, and focus on the entire experience of eating. Try to taste and smell what you're eating to get the most out of it.

"I try to spend five minutes after each meal just savouring the experience. I find that I enjoy the meal much more, and reach my satiety level."

Meg, age 44, 17 pounds lost

"I find if I talk a lot during my meal, I'm just not as satisfied. Sometimes I'm not even aware of what I ate, or how much I ate."

Rich, age 36, 20 pounds lost

"I have to put my fork down while I'm chewing, or I'll plough through much too quickly to enjoy what I'm eating."

Paul, age 49, 92 pounds lost

Yo Yo Dieting Is Not Dangerous

Even if you've been on a diet roller coaster for most of your life, it's less dangerous to your health to go up and down than it is to remain overweight. It doesn't hurt your metabolism, your cholesterol, or your blood pressure. It also doesn't make the pounds harder to budge.

"I can't believe that it took me seven tries to finally keep off that 40 pounds. Each time I tried, I would get within five pounds of my goal and gain it back. The first six times were expensive weight programmes, all of which you'd recognise. Only when I made up my own plan was I able to get it off and keep it off, which I've done for ten years."

Linda, age 50, 40 pounds lost

Make Sure You're Ready

Now may not be the right time to diet if:

1. When food comes up in a conversation, on TV, etc., it makes you hungry even if you've just eaten.

2. While losing weight, you constantly fantasise about your favourite foods.

15

3. While losing weight, your mood is one of anger and deprivation.

4. You expect to lose more than 3 to 4 pounds a week.

5. You cannot differentiate between physical and emotional hunger.

"My trigger food is pistachio ice cream. It's the one food that I crave, and causes me to break my diet. So before I finally lost the weight, I allowed myself a week of all the pistachio ice cream I wanted. I had to get it out of my system."

Chandra, age 26, 14 pounds lost

Prepare Yourself

Some of the biggest challenges to dieters are the social situations that crop up in everyday life. It is not practical to try to hide away from these events, so what can you do? Not to worry — simply preparing yourself for dining out, parties, family gatherings, etc., can keep you from breaking your diet. Watch out for the hidden calories and too much alcohol. For every glass of an alcoholic beverage you drink, accompany it with a glass of iced-water. This will keep you from becoming bloated, and will diffuse some of the effects. Choose fruit if you want dessert, or skip it altogether. If you do go off track, just get going again the next day.

"I always eat a light snack before I go to a party. Then I know I'll be in control when I get there."

Tammy, age 41, 13 pounds lost

"I wear the most body-revealing outfit I can find. When I was overweight I would purposely pick something loose so that I had room to eat. Knowing that what I'm wearing will not allow for bingeing keeps me in line."

Tina, age 33, 75 pounds lost

"I used to think about all the delicious food that was waiting for me at that special event. Now I go for the people."

Nick, age 67, 38 pounds lost

"My problem was the vending machine at the office. Now I make certain to bring a bag of carrots, and keep it right on top of my desk."

Wendy, age 32, 28 pounds lost

Seek Support

Find someone in your life you can commiserate with at least once a day. Feeling isolated can cause even the most determined dieter to fall off.

"I found a friend on the Internet who had a similar weight problem. We compared notes daily. Just writing to her made me feel better."

Polly, age 35, 68 pounds lost

"Making myself accountable to someone was as good for me as going to an expensive diet programme. At the end of each day, I called a friend who was known for her disciplined lifestyle and not only did she encourage me, but always had a new tip for my next day's challenge."

Sandy, age 25, 13 pounds lost

Organise Yourself

Too much free time on your hands can very often lead to mindless eating. On a sheet of paper, write out a daily schedule. Map out the time (in the beginning you'll need to do this by the half hour) and try to sneak in some activity. Note the dangerous spots of the day. For instance, if you tend to snack while waiting for dinner to cook, turn on the radio and dance around!

Count It Out

Silly as it sounds, this secret seems to work when you're enticed to reach for that tempting snack. Before you dig into that carton of ice cream, biscuit tin, etc., take a deep breath and count to 100. Usually, by the time you stop counting you will have convinced yourself that you don't really need it.

Use Lists

Shop with a list and you'll be less likely to compulsively pick things out, and end up with fattening goodies that will sabotage your efforts. You'll only gain a more expensive grocery tab, and you'll be missing things you need to keep on track.

Push Yourself

Only you can get yourself off the couch to exercise, cook that healthy dish, and move that body.

Why We Diet

67 per cent to be healthier
21 per cent to look better
6 per cent for a better love life
3 per cent for a better job
3 per cent just don't know

— from a survey by Johns Hopkins University

Maximise Your Breathing

The way you breathe can give you energy that you thought could only come from food. Many of us breathe shallowly through our mouths, which actually saps energy and keeps our body in a state of stress. Taking deep, slow, controlled breaths through your nose will get more air into your lungs and bloodstream. This will also cause waste products to be taken out of your body tissues more efficiently.

Don't Expect Too Much

Strange, isn't it, that we always want it all — and right now. Make certain that your expectations are reasonable. Expect to feel healthier, look better, and be more fabulous than you've ever been. If you expect that first, before expecting to reach that low mark on the scale, you're more likely to actually achieve it all.

"Deciding to let destiny guide my final outcome was a real 'freeing' experience for me. I made the decision to only put food into my body that would nurture it and help it run more efficiently. I let my body figure out what my weight should be, not some dumb chart."

Eva, age 34, 66 pounds lost

Learn to Enjoy Life

Get beyond the idea that your life is all about your weight and food. While you're losing weight, gain the pleasures of those physical, spiritual, and intellectual components that make you fully human.

Break Some Rules

Yes, most diets don't call for biscuits. But if a biscuit a day makes you feel like one of the living, go for it. It's your life, your body, and only you know what you need to get you through the day. Just remember that while one biscuit is fine, a whole packet will make you feel worse.

Chapter Two

Dieting Myths

Diet Supplements

You already know by now how dangerous prescription weight-loss supplements can be. Many over-the-counter supplements, if used inappropriately, can cause dizziness and other side effects.

Food Fakes

Frozen Yoghurt: Has less calcium and as much sugar as regular yoghurt, without the benefits of active cultures.

Sports Drinks: These highly acidic beverages contain lots of calories and can harm tooth enamel.

Fat-Free Pretzels: Don't bother — pretzels are already low in fat.

Low-Fat Biscuits: You'll end up eating too many, because the truth is they just don't satisfy.

Unrealistic Goals

Don't set yourself up for failure. You'll sabotage all your good efforts if you compare yourself to airbrushed models or professionally made-up movie stars.

Forgetting Calories

Believing the latest hype that it's fat grams that count, many dieters have found the weight just not moving, because they don't look at the calorie count of what they're eating. Remember, it's a combination of the two that will get you to your goal.

Money Doesn't Buy Motivation

Dieters have been fooled into spending large sums of money to enter a diet club or programme that promises to help you lose the weight. Remember, you are still the one doing the work, no matter how much you spend on some pricey gimmick.

"I became a diet club junkie, going from programme to programme. I'm sure that I spent thousands of pounds, believing that someone else was going to set me free from my years of overeating. It was only when I came to the decision to take charge of my own body that I dropped the pounds."

Dan, age 47, 130 pounds lost

"Boy, was I in the wrong place. I had only 15 pounds to lose, so I thought I would go to a weekly weigh-in to keep me honest. The lecturer was 25 pounds heavier than me, and then had the nerve to give me a goal that was totally unrealistic."

Sue, age 31, 16 pounds lost

Fasting

Although some dieters have had success with a one-day-a-week fruit "detox" diet, most reported that fasting only caused lightheadedness and deep feelings of deprivation.

Low Self-Esteem

A report by the University of Wisconsin-Madison cites that men and women with low self-esteem were more likely to be overweight, smoke, consume more alcohol, and expose themselves to dangerous situations.

"While losing the weight, I went into therapy. I realised I needed to fix my head while working on my body."

Marcie, age 28, 47 pounds lost

Believing Setbacks Are Fatal

Learning to accept setbacks as a part of being human will help you cause yourself less frustration on the road to success. Setbacks, when viewed as learning tools, actually help dieters achieve their final goals. Just about every person with a great body I've encountered has experienced a glitch somewhere in their attempt to slim down. Those who succeeded were able to step back, analyse what went wrong, correct the problem(s), and then use it as part of their motivation.

"When I started the final programme that became my final success, I took pen in hand and listed all the times I had tried to lose weight in my life, and what happened that made me get off track. What I found was that it was the same situation playing itself over and over again."

Chandra, age 51, 58 pounds lost

Not Setting Goals

Failure to set goals and a timetable throws the whole diet experience up in the air. While unrealistic goal setting (ten pounds in one week, five dress sizes by that reunion, etc.) can sabotage even the most determined dieter, there has to be some sort of pot at the end of the rainbow. Maybe your goal will be to drop a size by your birthday or learn a healthy way to fix your favourite dish. Make it a goal that will eventually get you to your long-awaited success.

"I found that mapping out a goal that had nothing and everything

23

to do with my weight loss was an important key in getting me back to the old me that I had lost. At the end of every month, I called an old friend. My weight had made me embarrassed to be seen, and as the weight came off, so did my shame."

Buck, age 42, 155 pounds lost

Fear of Judgement

Some dieters wouldn't leave their homes because they were so ashamed of their weight gain. They created a "Catch-22" situation — with the world revolving around them, they would sit home, consoling themselves with ice cream, chips, etc.

"While my girlfriends would go out on dates, I would stay home, sit on my couch and cry into my Chinese takeaway. Saturday nights were brutal! Becoming my own best friend, going to movies by myself (the biggest milestone), shopping alone, and seeking out others who were also 'dateless' took me out of my self-pitying mode that made things feel so much worse."

Felicia, age 25, 57 pounds lost

Bad Habits

List all those bad habits and change them into good ones.

"Believe me, I never thought that cleaning my plate was a bad habit, but when I was really full, I would continue to eat until everything was gone. Leaving food on my plate was hard to do, but helped me get my appetite back in check. But even today, I occasionally can hear my mother telling me about all the starving children who would be happy to have my food. Sorry, Mum, but it never made me happy to hear that."

Cassie, age 45, 69 pounds lost

Using Food to Rebuild Energy

Why is it when people are tired, they believe that only food will get them going again? The problem is that it's not so much that they eat, it's the foods they're choosing. Eating regularly is one of the best ways to keep energy high and fuel metabolic processes. However, choosing junk food as a quick fix will cause brain sugar to rise suddenly and then crash. It's a temporary fix that generally lasts no longer than an hour. While it's tempting to reach for a chocolate bar, fruit is absorbed more slowly into the body and will provide an even energy boost without the highs and lows of sugary snacks.

Here's another idea. When you get tired, rest! A cat nap is a no-calorie revitaliser!

Putting Yourself First

Believing that spending time on yourself is too self-indulgent only leads you on the road to failure. Taking time to become the best you can be allows you to give to others and feel good about doing it.

Not Understanding the Dynamics
The truth is that there are reasons lurking behind many weight problems. Yes, there are genetic components and family customs that may be responsible, but there also may be hidden sexual or physical abuse and other issues that no diet can cure. There is no diet that can cure emotional pain. Understanding this, perhaps including professional therapy, might be necessary before the real transformation can begin.

Refusing to Grow Up
Food cravings can be reminders of our childhood. Comfort foods are usually the foods that Mum made for you when you came home and it was cold, the school bully caught up with you, etc. These foods still feel good today. Researchers have found

that it isn't just taste, but the chemical reaction to the brain that makes these foods so appealing.

Believing It's Glandular

In only a very few instances is it true that weight problems are caused by the glands. But if this thinking is holding you back, go check it out with a doctor. Either way, you'll then be able to get on with a solution.

Limiting Cereals and Breads

Many believe that eliminating cereals and breads from their diet would help them achieve their goals. But the fact is that there's no one food that's bad for you. It's always a matter of quantity.

"I happen to adore bread. I love baking it, checking out ethnic bakeries, and the smell is heavenly! I also believe it's been a major player in my ongoing struggles with weight. I knew I'd never make it down the scale without bread. I kept it in my diet, but rather than slathering it in butter, jams, etc., I decided to eat the bread, and nothing else. I limited myself to two slices a day, and I made sure that I microwaved it. This way, the replete, just-baked taste made me feel absolutely decadent."

Maura, age 36, 32 pounds lost

"Sometimes I make cereal my supper. I like the fun of eating cereal, the fibre is good for me, and it usually is fairly high in protein. It has been essential in helping me with my final weight loss. Adding fruit makes it a complete meal."

Sue, age 27, 19 pounds lost

"I look for the low-fat breads now available at most natural supermarkets. They are surprisingly tasty, and contain lots of nutrients. Bread seems to calm me down and keep me feeling satisfied."

Mandy, age 33, 20 pounds lost

Bananas Are Fattening

Although a banana is sweeter than an apple or orange, it has only 85 calories. Bananas are a wonderful source of potassium and contain valuable protein. Dieters report bananas are more filling than some of the other fruits, and they're also great for alleviating constipation.

Exercising Is Dangerous During a Menstrual Cycle

Actually, women who exercise during their periods find that it helps to alleviate their cramps. Of course, it's important to listen to your body and only do what your body can.

Vitamins Give You Energy

There are a lot of people popping vitamins in the morning, believing that they're getting an energy boost for the day. The fact is that the energy you get is from the nutrients in the foods you eat. That's why it is important to put foods into your body that will provide you with the proper fuel to get through your day. Especially when you're dieting, it is important to choose foods which will provide the most power. But since you are most likely cutting down on what you eat, some supplementation is not a bad idea.

Chicken and Fish Are Lower in Cholesterol

The cholesterol content in chicken and fish is virtually the same as in other meats. However, poultry and fish do have a lower fat content than most red meat.

Losing Five Pounds Is No Big Deal

Oh, yeah? Take a five-pound bag of sugar and carry it around for an hour. Then you'll begin to appreciate those minor milestones of your weight loss. Every bit of weight you lose brings improved health and vitality.

Carbohydrates Make You Fat

Lately, just about every article or book around blames carbohydrates for all the problems of extra weight. Why blame carbohydrates? Because reducing fat and calories didn't work. Neither did reducing protein. So what else is left to blame? The truth is that researchers have found some serious problems with the oh-so-trendy high-protein diets of late. There is evidence that these diets are not very healthy and may lead to certain medical conditions. Plus, researchers point out that not all carbohydrates are the same.

Standing Up to Eat Will Burn More Calories

Not only is this dieting myth not true, but eating like this will cause you to overeat. You should never eat when standing up unless absolutely necessary.

Low-Fat Foods Are Low in Sugar

This myth has really helped the fat-free biscuit market. Unfortunately it's just not true. Simply because a food is low fat, doesn't mean it's necessarily healthy. These low-fat foods may be loaded with sugar, sodium, and chemical preservatives.

Natural Vitamins Are Better

Not only is this not true, but most of the time your body can't tell the difference between a vitamin from food or a test tube. In fact, scientists find that some "natural" vitamin sources contain higher levels of contaminants than more carefully refined ingredients used in the manufacturing process.

Grilled Vegetables Are Lower in Calories

The next time you're in a restaurant, I hope you will watch how grilled vegetables are cooked. They throw so much oil on them that the vegetables, especially the soft ones (zucchini, eggplant, mushrooms, etc.), just soak it up. This turns that grilled veggie dish into one of the heaviest entrees listed on a restaurant's menu!

Earrings to Control Cravings

There are a host of "magnetic wellness" products, one of which is an earring that allegedly controls appetite and cravings. The earrings supposedly work on the same premise as acupuncture. A part of the ear is related to hunger, and the earrings press on that spot to stop cravings. Quite a few of the more "desperate dieters" have tried these peculiar posts, and the only thing that stopped them from eating was that the pain they experienced wearing these earrings made it impossible to concentrate on anything else.

Subliminal Tapes

Lots of companies have come out with motivational tapes to lose weight. Success levels with them are questionable. In fact, one of my interviewees said that the voice on the tape was so annoying that the stress from listening to him drove her to the refrigerator.

Be Wary of Mr Muffin Man

Muffins are as different as Olympians and couch potatoes. While some are fairly healthy, like oat bran, others contain as many as 450 calories. Not only is it important to look for low-fat muffins and muffins rich in fibre, but also be sure to check calorie content. Some low fat-muffins contain as many calories as regular muffins because of added sugar.

Brown Sugar Is Better Than White

All brown sugar has over its white counterpart is a little bit of molasses. It is not nutritionally superior.

Spot Exercise Can Reduce Fatty Areas

While spot exercising can tighten muscle, it has no effect on fat.

Exercising in Special Sweats and Rubber Aids Fat Elimination

It seems to appear to work because you lose water through perspiration. However, the body will hang on to the fat, and the weight will come right back.

Margarine Is Better Than Butter

Here's the truth. Margarine is completely man-made and has absolutely no nutritional benefits. Butter is natural and has anti-cancer and anti-viral properties. There is research in its early stages that says butter may even help in the prevention and treatment of Alzheimer's disease. Unfortunately, some margarine has been linked with causing cancer. Butter contains the same amount of fat as margarine. Margarine's only benefit is that it contains no cholesterol, while butter contains about 12 grams per tablespoon. So do spread it sparingly.

Eliminate Eggs

Don't bother! Eggs have always been good for you. Eating eggs a couple of times a week as an entree will give you an excellent protein meal with few calories. Load up that omelette with lots of vegetables as a delicious diet tool.

Microwaves Destroy Vitamins

The opposite is true. Less vitamins are destroyed this way than in traditional ovens. Microwaves pass through your food without any harmful effects.

Nonfat Foods Are Healthiest

This is another long-held myth that has held us hostage from food enjoyment. Fat in food not only curbs hunger, but it helps

30

keep insulin levels steady.

Caffeinated Beverages Can Energise

These popular drinks have a dehydrating effect that can drain your energy. Coffee, tea and fizzy drinks are stimulants that bring you up quickly and then let you crash. It's important when drinking any caffeinated beverage to chase it with an equal amount of iced-water. It's also important to drink water with every alcoholic beverage, another dehydrator.

Saunas Can Help Shed Pounds

Although sitting in a sauna can feel great, any weight you lose is water weight. Once you replenish the fluids you've lost, the weight comes right back.

Fasting Eliminates Toxins

Each and every scientist I interviewed refuted any evidence that fasting eliminates toxins of any variety. Do it for religious reasons or to protest nuclear waste sites, but your body naturally eliminates unwanted substances through the usual waste processes.

Form Doesn't Matter When Exercising

Weight training and cardiovascular workouts can backfire if you're doing them wrong because you may end up working a different muscle than intended. Worse, you can put unnecessary stress on your joints.

"I thought I would try to exercise from some charts I found in a magazine. I ended up doing it wrong, and bulked up in the area I had hoped to slim."

Jerry, age 25, 32 pounds lost

Taste Bud Inhibitor

This is an orthodontically fitted mouth piece that covers the taste buds on the roof of your mouth so that you can't enjoy the taste of food. It costs about £180 and requires a dentist to fit it properly. Save your money. Taste is not the only reason we eat.

Fibre Tablets

The problem with these tablets is that they don't provide the variety of fibre that you get with natural fibre. If you're looking for a fibre supplement to add to your diet, try the liquid fibre supplements available at most drugstores. Better yet, choose a breakfast cereal with at least six grams of fibre. That should do it.

Corsets for Weight Contouring

Women all over the country are picking up on the new undergarments that hearken back to the Victorian era. Today's corsets allege to celebrate the female form, when in fact they are reviving the barbaric practices of the past. Some women are corseting themselves as a way to control their eating. They can only digest fruits and grains — pizza would be prohibitive. Physicians report that some of the dangers of corseting include muscle atrophy (the body stops relying on natural muscle), aching kidneys, digestive problems, and unhealthy pressure on the organs. It can also interrupt breathing and even hinder menstrual cycles.

Lack of Time

With grocery aisles full of healthy packaged foods, it can't get much easier, no matter how little time you have to cook, to stay on track with your diet. Make up your menus ahead of time, and stock up on low-fat packaged foods so when you come home stressed out, wanting that quick fix, you'll have a variety of meals ready to cater to your taste at the time. Ideally you should be able to combine a packaged food with something fresh. Happily, fresh foods are also becoming more convenient, like cut-up salad mixes. Meat also comes cut-up, and vegetables now come peeled and sliced too. And don't forget breakfast foods for a quick, satisfying meal any time of day.

Alcohol and Diets Don't Mix

Although alcohol contains calories, there are low-calorie choices. Champagne and wine spritzers top the list. If your lifestyle has always allowed for social drinking, there is no reason to stop. Just stay away from the eggnog and that occasional drink will blend right into your weight-loss efforts. According to the American Cancer Society, active women who walked at least four hours a week, ate a vegetable-rich diet, and had a glass of wine or beer with dinner up to five nights a week lost more abdominal weight than healthy, active nondrinkers.

Overdoing and Rushing Your Programme

You'll burn out faster than a match in a wind tunnel if you try to do it all at once. Not only that, you could cause yourself serious health damage short- and long-term.

The Diet Shot

Some alternative diet doctors are administering injections of adrenal cortex extract. The highly controversial extract is taken from the adrenal glands of cattle, sheep and other animals. The concept is that the injection will help ease a dieter's salt cravings and regulate their blood pressure. There is no research proving these benefits, and there have been bacterial infections involved. The Food and Drug Administration has issued alerts and warnings of serious, life-threatening injuries associated with such shots.

Trying to Look Like Barbie, Today's Supermodels, and Mannequins

Yes, there are some women who are having plastic surgery to look like this physically impossible childhood creature, but it just can't be done. Not only are Barbie's vital statistics physiologically impossible, her neck is twice the length of that of a normal human being.

The typical model weighs 20 per cent less than the average woman. Just ten years ago, she weighed 8 to 10 percent less.

The vital statistics of store mannequins are so extreme that if a woman tried to equate their shape, she would not have enough body fat to menstruate.

Fast Music Eating

Listening to your favourite dance tune while you're eating will get your mouth moving and plate clean in record time. There have been numerous studies that suggest that people who listen to fast music while dining will take more and larger forkfuls of food per minute than those who listen to slow music. Those doo-wopping diners took an average five forkfuls per minute while the slow dancers, or no-music diners, took only three. The fast music diners also were more apt to ask for seconds. The reason you need to slow your eating down is that the brain needs to register that it's full, and once it does, you consume less.

Bright Colours

"Hot" colours, including red, orange, and yellow, stimulate your mood and your appetite. That's bad news if you're trying to cut down. That's why McDonald's (yellow arches) and other fast food chains use these colours to their advantage. Make certain that the dishes you use are either clear, white, or pastel, and that your dining area is decorated in soft tones.

Boredom

Make sure that there's enough variety in your diet, workouts, and your life. More dieters went off their diets because of the sheer tedium than for any other reason.

Basing Worth on Weight

Feeling that you need to be the skinniest belle of the ball may mean that you have serious esteem issues that no diet can cure.

"Every morning my mood would be decided by my weight. If I was a pound or two down, I was absolutely up, on a real high. If the scale showed a higher number than the previous day, I was impossible to be around. I finally had to throw away my scales until I got myself straight. Now, I've reincorporated the scales into my weight management, but I only allow myself to use it once a week."

Vicki, age 38, 45 pounds lost

Too Little Calories

Consume enough to fuel your body, but not so many that they get stored as fat. Skip "empty" calories with no nutritional value.

Energy Bars

Only use these convenience bars in an emergency. Don't use them as meal replacements. They contain too many calories for the little satisfaction that they provide. They really are intended for professional athletes, and somehow have made their way over to the diet population.

Skipping Breakfast

Your body has been on an 8- to 12-hour fast. It needs fuel. You'll only make up for it later.

Chapter Three

Food Choices

You Should Eat

First, the good news. Severe rationing of calories in a diet makes it harder, rather than easier, to lose weight. Dieters who eat more of low-fat foods lose weight more efficiently than those who eat lower-calorie menus with more fat. Eating the right foods can actually boost your body's ability to burn fat. Also, studies done on drastic weight-loss programmes have proven that decreased brain function and reaction time are consequences of such a dramatic change.

What Should I Eat?

Topping your list of foods to include on your diet should be those that stimulate the body to lose weight. These include:

Grains: pasta, oatmeal, corn, pretzels, popcorn, rice

Fruits: apples, cherries, oranges, grapefruit, bananas

Vegetables: broccoli, spinach, carrots, green beans

Great Munchies

Don't think twice about these snacks. You can munch away and still lose the pounds. With these foods, you almost burn more calories chewing and digesting them than they actually contain.

Under 20 Calories

8oz courgette sticks — 18 calories
8oz cucumber slices — 13 calories
4oz pickled vegetables (giardiniera) — 10 calories
2 tablespoons of salsa — 20 calories
Diet ice lolly — 10 calories
1 dill pickle — 12 calories

Under 50 Calories

10 jelly beans — 40 calories
20 raisins — 35 calories
1 small peach — 35 calories
8 baby carrots — 32 calories
8oz popcorn (air-popped) — 30 calories
8fl oz tomato juice — 41 calories
8oz strawberries — 43 calories
Nonfat cappuccino — 43 calories

Fast Food Facts

Eating on the road can play havoc with even the best-laid dieting plans. Order grilled rather than fried, avoid fattening dressings, and go for small-size servings.

Subway has a sandwich called the Veggie Delite. At just 237 calories and 3 grams of fat, it's a great way to eat on the run.

Kentucky Fried Chicken features Red Beans and Rice at just 126 calories and 4 grams of fat.

Dairy Queen's DQ Sandwich is just 140 calories and 4 grams of fat.

Burger King's Chunky Chicken Salad is only 142 calories and 4 grams of fat.

Arby's Roast Chicken Salad is 149 calories and 2 grams of fat.

McDonald's features Grilled Chicken Salad Deluxe. It's a great choice at just 120 calories and under 2 grams of fat.

McDonald's McGrilled Chicken Classic has 260 calories and just 4 grams of fat.

Wendy's sour cream and chive baked potato contains 80 calories and 6 grams of fat.

Steam it Up

For added nutrition, steam your vegetables. Boiling destroys vitamins. Microwaving vegetables is also preferable to boiling them.

Eat Pasta

Pasta is a highly satisfying food that won't put weight on you as long as it's not swimming in sauce. It's easy to cook and store, and can be used in a variety of dishes. Since it contains mostly starch, it also slowly rations out energy. It's one of the slowest-burning foods.

Eat Soup

Start a meal with soup or use it as a nutritious snack and you'll stave off hunger pangs. Tomato soup, made with water, contains just 85 calories a cup. Throw in some vegetables for vitamins, a few beans for fibre, and you've got a nutritious meal.

Make It Spicy

Not only do spices make low-fat foods more desirable and satisfying, they also rev up the metabolism. Start a collection of dried and fresh herbs and spices.

Easy Substitutions

Instead of cream use evaporated skimmed milk or yoghurt.

Apple sauce holds moisture in. Use it when a recipe calls for oil or butter.

When a recipe calls for sugar, taking as much as 25 per cent out will not affect taste.

Sprinkle powdered sugar over pancakes instead of syrup.

Spread your bagel with low-fat jam instead of cream cheese.

Use mustard instead of mayonnaise in your sandwiches.

Use wine vinegar instead of vinaigrette in your salad.

Top a baked potato with salsa in place of butter.

Ice a cake with marshmallow creme instead of icing.

Drink Your Coffee

No matter how hard they try, scientists can't prove that coffee does any real harm. There are even recent studies that indicate that drinking fresh brewed coffee can up your antioxidant quotient.

Fill Up on Celery

Because it takes up so much space in your stomach, celery is the snack choice of the world's most beautiful bodies. It's a great source of fibre and a natural cure for constipation. It also contains both calcium and magnesium.

Choose Cereals for Fibre Content

Not all cereals are created equal. Choose cereals with at least 5 grams of fibre. Good choices include: Shredded Wheat, Grape-Nuts, Raisin Bran, and Muesli. There are several others. Also be aware of calorie content. It varies greatly between cereals and brands.

The best thing about cereals is that some super-fortified varieties contain 100 per cent of the Recommended Daily Allowance (RDA) for many vitamins and minerals. If you eat on the run, or skip meals, these cereals are an important source of nutrients.

"I eat my cereal as a snack, a quick dinner, and often carry sandwich bags of it in my car. I find it a filling, rewarding treat. It's fun to try the different varieties. It breaks up the monotony of getting in my fibre. I even treat myself to the occasional sugary children's cereals."

Mary, age 48, 33 pounds lost

Select the Right Cut of Meat
The fat content in meats varies from 1 per cent for 4 ounces of skinless turkey breast to 9 per cent for 4 ounces of beef sirloin. Allow for this when planning out your meals.

4 ounces of:
Skinless chicken breast has 4 grams of fat
Beef medallion has 5 grams of fat
Pork tenderloin has 7 grams of fat
Pork chop has 8 grams of fat
Lamb shank has 8 grams of fat

One pound of fat is 3,500 calories.

Good Eggs
A large egg has only 75 calories and 1.6 grams of fat. Use eggs as an inexpensive source of protein. After years of getting a bad rap, the poor egg is finally off the diet hit list. Plus, eggs are an important source of vitamin K, selenium, and riboflavin.

Foods for Good Looks
You are what you eat, no doubt about it. Why not let your diet nourish your looks as well as your body?

Sweet Potatoes: Vitamin A is known to be a remarkable antiwrinkling agent. Sweet potatoes are full of this important vitamin. The pleasing result is clearer, smoother skin.

Wheat Germ: If you want to get rid of pimples quickly and efficiently, make sure to include two or three tablespoons a day in your diet. Add it to cereal, yoghurt, and cottage cheese.

Cheese: To ensure a happy smile, add a slice or two of hard cheese into your diet. Choose Swiss, cheddar, or gouda to block bacteria in the mouth and prevent cavities.

Satisfy Your Cravings

Want to crunch? Choose pretzels or pita chips. Need something smooth and comforting? Low-fat puddings or frozen fruit lollies are ideal.

Don't Bother!

Although it's important to eliminate fat in our diets, don't worry about taking out whole milk from coffee. You only save about four calories, and many dieters believe that skimmed milk makes their coffee taste too watery.

All Lettuce Is Not Created Equal

Choose colour when it comes to salad fixings. The darker the colour, the more vitamins and minerals. Butter head, Romaine, and loose-leaf contain larger amounts of iron than the typical iceberg salad lettuce.

Dessert Ideas You'll Really Use!

Put whipped cream on top of sugar-free jelly. It tastes sinful, and will add only 8 calories with a single gram of fat.

Combine orange marmalade with orange liqueur. Drizzle over orange slices. Dollop with whipped cream.

Core but don't peel an apple. Dust inside with cloves, cinnamon, and a little brown sugar. Bake for 30 minutes at 375 degrees farenheit.

Pop some popcorn and spray with a little nonfat butter spray. Sprinkle with cinnamon and a packet of sugar substitute.

Break Your Bread
Cut your pizza into little pieces and tear up your bread. The value of cutting your food into smaller portions lies in making your food last longer so you're satisfied with less. Dipping your bread into salad dressing, sour cream, and other condiments works the same way.

Prevent Bottom Feeding
Sitting down in certain places signals us that it's time to eat. Trigger areas include the couch in front of the TV, cinemas, sporting events, or your mother's kitchen table. Even cars can be culprits. Get a motivational tape to play while you drive. Chew some gum while watching TV. Hold your partner's hand in the cinema. Make alternative plans when you know your hunger will be triggered.

What to Eat Each Day?
You should choose foods that you enjoy, of course, but you need to include the following:

Vegetables:
Three to five servings. Try to include one serving of raw, leafy greens.

Meat:
Have no more than three 3-ounce servings a day. Cut off all fat. Try to make two servings of turkey or chicken. One serving of fish a day is ideal.

Fruits:

2 to 3 servings daily. One-half cup of chopped or sliced fruit is a serving.

Dairy:

At least two servings daily. A serving would be 8 ounces of milk or yoghurt. 1½ ounces of cheese is a serving.

Fats

Salad dressing, cooking oil, butter, and mayonnaise should be limited to 2 servings a day.

How Big Is a Portion?

Trying to figure out what is the right amount to eat during a diet can become a challenge and an annoyance. Of course, you're not about to bring out the diet scales at the table in order to figure your portion size. However, your hand can tell you all you need to know. Your palm is the size of a 3-ounce portion of meat. Your fist is a cup, while your thumb is just about right for one ounce.

Stretch Out High-Calorie Foods

Use low-calorie fillers in dishes that pack a lot of calories. You'll still get the taste and satisfaction. For instance, add an extra portion of steamed rice to Chinese dishes. Double the lettuce and tomato in a sandwich. Add some sprouts to your potato salad.

"I look for fruits that have a high water content, and never eat any fruits that contain a lot of sugar. I'm trying to lose my sweet tooth. I'm also staying away from grapes because they are higher in calories and I tend to lose count."

Rachel, age 24, 14 pounds lost

"Whenever I eat fruit, I keep the stone in my mouth for about fifteen minutes. Sucking on the stone keeps the flavour in my mouth, and makes me think I'm still enjoying the fruit."

Genna, age 28, 26 pounds lost

"I need to fool myself a lot in order to stay on my diet. I grate almost everything I eat. This includes carrots, cabbage, and even apples. It gives me so much more volume. Sometimes I mix the carrots, cabbage, and apples together with a little vinegar and mayonnaise for an enormous coleslaw!"

Jinks, age 31, 20 pounds lost

"I love the taste of almonds. I use low-calorie almond extract on fruits, cottage cheese, yoghurt, even in water. It tastes absolutely sinful with no added calories. Flavour is everything to me."

Mona, age 61, 33 pounds lost

Chapter Four

Looking Good While Slimming Down

Dress Up for a New You

Don't wait until you've lost the weight to start to care about your appearance. Do it now, while you keep going down. You will not only look more attractive, but you'll feel so much better about yourself.

Rules of Dressing Thinner

1. Match your tights to your shoes. Legs look longer and thinner when your tights are toned to skirts and shoes.

2. Pleated trousers conceal tummy bulges, so if this is your problem use those pleats to your advantage. The pleats must not be too full, though.

3. An A-line skirt can emphasise body length while hiding heavy thighs.

4. Use a shirt like a jacket or a tunic. Choose a generously cut shirt in a heavy or lined fabric. It's an elegant look over slim pants, flowing over every possible sin.

5. Dress in one colour. Wearing one colour from shoulder to shoe streamlines the body. It's called monochromatic dressing. If you don't want to limit yourself to just one colour, choose colours that are closely matched. If you really want to go for "thin" stick to darker colours.

6. If you have a chubby neck, choose v-necklines. They create the illusion of a longer, leaner body.

7. To bring attention to the face, and away from the body, wear a choker and matching earrings.

8. A long jacket is a "pounds parer". It can make any outfit look elegant while hiding figure flaws.

9. Choose a low-heeled shoe that is cut low on the instep. Stick to a thinner, more graceful heel.

10. A loosely fitted waistcoat can hide a thick waist.

11. Wear belts in a low-slung manner, or gently held around the waist.

12. Always wear control top tights with Lycra.

13. A body suit can eliminate bulge. It also gets rid of unsightly "panty line" and fabric pulling.

14. Choose a well-fitted jacket. A look that is too loose or boxy tends to add pounds.

15. Simple styling is most slimming. Cuffs, pockets, and buttons can add width to the body.

16. Wear prints only at the slimmest part of your body. Stay with smaller prints, rather than big flowery ones. Florals have direction like any other print. Look for designs with vertical or diagonal movement.

17. Look for fabrics that drape the body. This would include light woollens, cotton and rayon.

18. Stay away from very large shoulder pads. They may seem to add balance, but they're really only adding bulk.

19. Double breasted and breast pockets should be avoided if you're top heavy.

20. Lightweight knits can be slimming, if not worn too tight to the body. Let it skim the body, rather than cling to it.

21. Choose sturdy shoes, even heels. Delicate shoes make thick ankles look thicker.

22. A sarong skirt tied in front hides a tummy.

23. A shorter length makes for a leggier look.

24. A gently nipped-in waist trims the middle of the body.

25. Vertical buttons and seams lengthen the torso area.

> Stand Tall! You'll look thinner, more confident, and more attractive with good posture.

Hair-Styling Tricks

A good stylist can take pounds off your face with the right haircut.

Layers are the most important tool a stylist can use in slenderising the face. Full cheeks become sculpted by creating angles starting at the temple and ending just below the cheekbones.

A **round face** can be lengthened by creating a wispy fringe cut in an upside down "v" pattern. The shortest section of the fringe will be at the centre of the forehead.

Double chins can be easily camouflaged by beginning layering at the jawbone just below the earlobe. Finish laycring just below the chin.

Blow drying hair on a large round brush directly on to the face reduces width, frames your best features, and is extremely sexy.

An elegantly **upswept hairdo** with loosely gathered tendrils around the face brings attention away from the body.

Highlights create long vertical lines and the illusion of slimness.

Height in the crown of the head will instantly lengthen the face.

Consider **lightening** your hair by a shade or two. It will open up the face, and instantly slim down cheekbones.

> "The bigger the hair the smaller the hips."
> Fran Drescher

Bronzing Powder — A Dieter's Best Friend

Looking to slim down your face with makeup? Head to your local drugstore and pick up an inexpensive bronzing powder. Use it to slim down your nose by running it down the sides. Create the illusion of cheekbones in a much more subtle and believable way by running the bronzer under the cheekbone area. Disguise a double chin by running the bronzer under the jaw line. Can't find any bronzing powder? Choose face powder in a colour two shades darker than your foundation.

Other Makeup Tips

Highlight Your Chin, Forehead, Nose Bridge, and Brow Bone

Dust a translucent face powder over the tip of your chin to emphasise its length. Use over the nose to focus the attention on the top of the nose, rather than the sides. Bring attention to the outside of the eyes by sweeping powder just below the outer portion of the eyebrow arch.

Play Up Your Brows

Bringing attention to your eyebrows will take focus away from that double chin, puffy cheeks, etc. The brow is known as the "frame for the face". Darken your brow a bit, eliminate any stray hairs, and be sure to brush upwards. Keep your brows in place with a bit of hairspray. Spray it on an old toothbrush (or even on your index finger).

Emphasise Your Eyes
Line the lower rim of your lids with a white pencil. Curl upper lashes with an eyelash curler. Apply at least two coats of mascara to the upper lashes only. Apply shadow only at the outer corners of the eye in the shape of a sideways "v".

Elongate Your Hands
Little tricks you can use on your nails will benefit in your hands looking longer and thinner. Switch to a lighter shade of nail polish. Stay with beige and pink tones, so that they will blend right into your skin. If your nails are short, lengthen them by applying polish only on the centre portion of the nail. Leave a sliver of bare nail on either side.

Fake a Good Body
Male and female models do it all the time. They work their muscles just before a photo shoot. If you have an event coming up, don't panic! You too can create a temporary "pumped" look. Here are some things that you can do just before going out so that you can really look good in that body-revealing outfit.

1. Holding a ten-pound weight, slowly lift it up and out to the side, bending arm at elbow. Slowly lower.

2. Holding a ten- or twenty-pound weight behind the head with both hands, slowly lower hands to the middle of the back. Be sure to hold elbows close to the head. Repeat 20 times.

3. You CAN wear that backless dress. Lift your arms straight out to the sides and squeeze shoulder blades toward each other. Count to ten and release. Do this at least 15 times. Holding 5- to 10-pound weights will yield optimum results.

4. Fake long sleek legs by raising up on tiptoes for as long as

you can. Try to go a full minute. Raise up and down quickly. This will give your calves a firmer, more toned appearance.

5. Wear the highest heels you can walk in without killing yourself.

6. Hit the shower with a moisturising body exfoliator to slough off dead skin on arms and elbows.

7. Shave with a moisturising cream to avoid nicks.

8. Cover blemishes with a good concealer even on your shoulders and back.

9. Fake cleavage by dipping a brush into bronzing powder and dusting a half moon contour on each breast. Start from above the breastbone, and go over and up to the armpit. Do this very subtly and no one will ever know.

10. Apply a self-tanner all over your body.

Beat the Bloat

Use these model's tips to look more svelte in even the most body-revealing clothing.

1. Never drink from a straw, and never chew gum. Both will send air right to your tummy and distend and bloat you.

2. Avoid starches like pasta and bread. These foods cause the body to produce excess insulin, which puffs you out.

3. Eliminate salt for at least twelve hours before putting on anything body revealing.

4. Eat a few bites of protein. Turkey and fish are excellent choices for energy, and they'll keep you bright and wary of the fattening stuff.

5. Don't drink soda, not even diet. Doing so will give you a false, "fatter" body fat reading. The reason is, that it puffs up your body temporarily, even though there are no calories. It's the sodium that causes you to retain fluid responsible for this condition.

6. Rush blood to specific body areas for a more defined appearance.

    A. Balancing on your knees, squatting on the floor, lift your arms to your ears and then lower to your sides in one controlled movement. Do 3 sets of 10 each.

    B. Lie down with your legs raised in the air, knees slightly bent. Tuck your hands behind your head. Slowly lift your buttocks a few inches off the ground, squeezing them together as you lift. Hold to a count of 20. Lower slowly. Do this at least 25 times.

    C. Hold on to the back of a chair, legs spread apart, and toes pointed out. Squat until your thighs are parallel with your feet. Do this 30 times.

Swim Wear

Primal fear

I have heard more primal screaming coming out of dressing rooms at swimsuit time than at any other time of the year. It doesn't matter what size you are or what age — does not matter at all! Trying on swim wear has to rate right along with the stirrups in those doctor's offices. I'm not saying that buying a swimsuit will ever be fun, fun, fun, but I can make it a little less painful for you. Here goes:

Rule #1: Go Up a Size

This is not what most women want to hear, but because swimsuits are made of less fabric than other garments, they tend to run a bit smaller than normal street clothing. A size 12 suit will be very snug on a woman who wears a size 12 dress, but will be perfect on a woman who wears a size 10. If you insist on trying on your normal size, be certain that you can bend, stretch, sit, etc. without any discomfort or riding up.

Rule #2: Look at Tags

Thank the designer gods for finally listening to us. They have developed swim wear that actually gives off the illusion of having lost ten pounds. You'll see it in the tag — usually these suits are called "minimisers". Again, try them on, because you may find them quite confining. It's nice to be tucked in, but who wants to feel that they're wearing a girdle on the beach?

Rule #3: Don't Be Afraid of Colour

There is no reason to stick to black or navy if you're trying to give off the illusion of slimness. Although darker colours do slim the body, vibrant shades like purple, magenta, maroon, and green also serve this purpose. You can also use colour to accentuate the positive, while hiding any negatives. For instance, if you want to show off a terrific bosom, choose a bright colour in the bodice area with a darker bottom. Don't be afraid of lines in the fabric. Vertical lines can be especially flattering, as well as geometric shapes and polka dots. They cause people's eyes to never rest on a specific body area. Patterns keep the eye moving.

Get Rid of That Big Handbag

Nothing ruins the look of a streamlined body more than a big old cluttered handbag. Take all the junk out, and throw away any bag larger than 10 by 13 inches. This is especially important for large-breasted women who look totally top heavy with an oversized handbag.

You Can Wear Shorts

They just have to be the right style. Sorry, no "Daisy Dukes" for you if you're not in perfect shape. Drawstring shorts can make heavy thighs look slimmer, and reduce down any waist. Pleated shorts slim down a puffy tummy and offer a longer line. Cigarette and Capri shorts instantly make your legs look long and lean. Chubby knees look great in the new just below the knee pedal-pusher styles. Walking shorts with a wide waistband actually raise your waist.

Help for Pear Shapes

Pear-shaped bodies are heavier below the waist, just like the fruit. The way to balance this figure type is to pad on top.

1. Look for bosom-maximixing details like epaulettes, breast pockets, and large buttons and embellishments.

2. Look for Empire styles.

3. Layer a shirt or sweater over a T-shirt or turtleneck.

Help for Apples

This body type (large torso and breasts with thin legs) needs help minimising the bust line.

1. Make sure that the shirt is fitting without gapping. An oversized shirt will only cause you to look even bulkier.

2. Choose a long pendant to lengthen the torso.

3. A V-neck will elongate and slim.

4. Choose a top that hits the hipbone. Stay away from tucked-in styles.

Looking Leggy

Legginess is in the eye of the beholder. There are easy ways to fake the look even if legs are not your strong point.

1. Wear a front-slit skirt. If you can carry off a long length, it will

be even more leg lengthening.

2. Match footwear, tights, and skirt.

3. Wear opaque tights with short skirts.

4. Wear some kind of heel, even with pants. Remember, the more casual the look, the thicker the heel. Flat heels squish you like a bug.

5. Always choose slim pants over flared or palazzo styling.

6. Wear long boots if you've got thick calves and ankles.

7. Choose a pencil skirt over a full dirndl type.

8. Never wear shiny or textured tights.

9. Stay away from straps.

10. Don't even think about socks, even with pants.

Large-Sized Fashion Mistakes

Pleated skirts

Fabric without substance

Large patterns

Accessories that are too dainty

Teeny tiny handbags

Clingy fabrics

Frilly silly clothing (stick with classics)

Use Body Shapers

The right lingerie can slim and tone you in all the right places. It gives your body a new look before you even begin losing the weight. While you're going down, it can keep loose skin streamlined instantly!

Some Choices:

Power slips

Uplift shapers

Slimming tights

Tummy-toning knickers

Have It Tailored

As you head down the scale, you'll find your clothes sizes changing quickly. Some things in your closet might be worth saving if you can find a good tailor or seamstress. Consider the costs.

Trousers hemmed: £12 to £15

Sleeves hemmed: £18 to £22

Skirts hemmed: £22 to £30

Shoulders taken in: £65 to £70

Waist taken in: £15 to £20

Tapering jacket, pants, or skirt: £22 and up

Maybe You Should Throw Those Big Clothes Away

If this is it, and you're definitely going to keep it off this time, consider giving away your large-sized clothing as soon as they become too big. Telling yourself that they may come in handy one day will become a self-fulfilling prophecy. Don't do that to yourself. They will become a huge albatross around your neck.

Buy Them a Little Too Small

Purchasing just one or two things that are a little bit too snug on you will be the perfect motivator to keep going on your weight-loss plan. You can hardly wait to get into them! But don't go crazy. You don't know for certain just where you'll end up, and those too-tight outfits could become too loose in a matter of a month or two. Dieters have told me that they underestimated their ability to lose weight, and wasted far too much money on "in-between" clothing.

Dress to Express

As your body comes out of hiding, so does your personality. Let your clothes and accessories give the image that you want out there. What do you want to say to people? Make certain the image that is out there is one that people will respect and admire. So maybe you're not feeling terribly good about your body right now. There's no need to shout that message out to the world. Dress as if you are feeling proud of yourself, and before you know it, you will be. Just keep faking it until you're finally feeling it.

Chapter Five

Secrets of Models and Celebrities

How Do They Stay So Thin?

Whenever anyone hears that I have been in the modelling profession for over 30 years and worked with the world's most glamorous celebrities, they always have questions. Surprisingly, the number one question I am asked is not "are they as nice or attractive in person?" Instead, everybody wants to know how models and superstars keep their bodies in such fabulous shape.

Are they born that way? No, not necessarily. What do they do? What's the big secret to their incredible shapes? The fact is that models and celebrities are just people. Yes, they are lovely-looking people, but believe it or not, they have the very same problems that everyone has. Yes, they even have weight problems. The difference is their looks have become their fortune, so they have pulled every trick in the book to get thin and stay there. Their livelihood depends on it.

Iced Water

You've heard that models drink lots of water. Well, that's very true, but it's only half the story. To get optimum benefits from water, models drink iced water. With iced water, the body needs to use over 40 calories just to warm itself to room temperature in order to absorb the water into the system. That means that the theory of negative calories is true. You are actually using more calories than

59

you are taking in.

Unfiltered Apple Cider Vinegar

What a versatile product! It's a great blood purifier when you put a tablespoon in a cup of hot water and drink it. You can also use it as an astringent for both your face and hair.

Colon Cleanser

No, I don't need to elaborate, but there is something to be said for the fact that if beauty is to really work, it needs to start from the "inside". Top actresses and great beauties throughout history have used this as an unconventional beauty/health regime. Legendary actress Mae West was famous for her daily enemas. Her skin was known to be as "soft as a baby's bottom" right up until the time of her death. These cleansers are now extremely popular, and readily available at health food stores in kits and capsules.

Kelp

Models carry kelp tablets to speed up their metabolism.

Dandelion Tea

This is used as a diuretic. Find this product in natural supermarkets and drugstores. Do stay near a bathroom. Sometimes it works rather quickly.

Top Models Must Stay in Top Form

Cindy Crawford tends to gain weight in the buttocks area. That's one reason why she reportedly avoids dairy products. She has stayed at the top of her field because she treats her body as a direct reflection of her success.

Niki Taylor gained a self-admitted 70 pounds during her pregnancy, going from a size 6 to a 20. With self-determination and discipline, she lost it all, and was back on the catwalk after only 3 months. Niki is an avid runner, and is known to favour a mostly vegetable diet devoid of any dressings or sauces.

Jelly Beans

A jelly bean is a quick energy boost, and surprisingly low in calories and fat. Most of these little treats contain only 5 or 6 calories each. Compared with a LifeSaver (10 calories), or stick of gum (up to 20 calories), it's a pretty good way to snack. Models always keep these in their bags.

Eating just twice a day is a fact of life for many models, including **Elle Macpherson**. Each day it's a choice between lunch or dinner, depending on her schedule or mood. Those incredible abs of hers are a result of 500 daily sit-ups.

Her legs are the longest in the business, and her diet is varied, but disciplined. **Nadja Auermann** is the German beauty designers usually book first to show off their seasonal collections. She is a known vegetarian, and like so many in her league, uses beans in place of meats in order to get enough protein in her diet.

Claudia Schiffer is yet another model who eats lightly at dinner (salad and steamed vegetables), and eats nothing but fruits before noon. She is often seen on location snacking on tomato juice, black grapes, and herbal tea. While some of her fellow models prefer to engage in heavy exercise to stay in shape, Claudia prefers to stay slim with a stringent diet plan.

Her disdain for exercise has been a problem for model turned TV host **Daisy Fuentes**. In the past, her weight has fluctuated greatly and been noticed by critics. But giving up her favourites, pizza and hamburgers, and joining a health club, have been the answer to finally arriving at a lean, stable weight.

Few models have remained in the business longer that **Lauren Hutton**. No exercise fanatic, Lauren prefers taking long walks instead. She claims that water is her biggest secret to a youthful body. She drinks it all day, while basing her diet around salads, fruits, and vegetables. She rarely eats meats or desserts.

Few people know that **Linda Evangelista** is a great cook who makes delicious low-fat dishes with creative substitutions. The only cravings she has are for meat, and she does allow herself an occasional hamburger. Since she is still actively modelling in her thirties, she is often seen at gyms pumping up her heart rate and toning her muscles on the treadmill and bicycle.

Beauty Has Never Been One Size Fits All

Audrey Hepburn was 5´7´´ and weighed just 110 pounds. She was out of sync with the other screen stars of her time like curvy Marilyn Monroe, Jane Russell, and Jayne Mansfield.

A Childhood Weight Problem

Ellen star **Joely Fisher**, daughter of Connie Stevens and Eddie Fisher, was overweight growing up, carrying an extra 35 pounds and the legacy of a drop-dead gorgeous mum, Joely keeps her weight off by getting out in nature and hiking hills. She's come a long way since the days she was known as "Roly Poly Joely". Here's Joely's favourite method for getting 5 pounds off fast! Joely advises to stay on this diet for no longer than a week:

Breakfast: Low-fat yoghurt and strawberries

Lunch & Dinner: Brown rice

Bulimia

Singer **Marie Osmond** has battled bulimia since she was a teenager. Although now living a healthy lifestyle, she confesses that she constantly battles the disease. She occasionally falls victim to a binge, eating an entire box of chocolates. She credits balance in her life, a supportive relationship with her husband Brian, and designing dolls (sold on QVC Shopping Network) for keeping her on track.

How Do They Stay So Slim?

Actress **Minnie Driver** relies on spirituality. She has been able to conquer a 30-pound weight gain and self-loathing to become one of the best success stories (and bodies) in Hollywood.

Ashley Judd maintains her 5'7", 125-pound figure with a heavy vegetable diet and by staying away from dairy foods. She begins her day with a drink of hot water and lemon, relies on herbs, and uses soy milk in her cereal. This southern belle grew up on fried chicken and biscuits, and still loves to bake.

Penelope Ann Miller makes sure she always fits exercise into her schedule, even when there's no gym available. While filming *Little City* she took the lift in her hotel to the 15th floor and walked to the 26th floor where she was staying. Rather than being driven to her trailer during breaks, she chose to walk (up to 20 times a day!). Adjusting her diet of skipping breakfast and eating a large dinner, she's changed her ways. Now she starts the day with a protein shake with nonfat milk and snacks on yoghurt and fruit.

Demi Moore got into shape for *Striptease* by enlisting the advice of topless dancers. She used combinations of stomach crunches, walking lunges, and leg lifts. Demi keeps her system cleaned out by drinking herb teas and vitamins. "Having the tea between meals fills me up while the vitamins keep me going."

Baywatch babe **Gena Lee Nolin** lost her pregnancy weight by replacing starches with produce. She began eating mini-meals 5 or 6 times a day in order to keep up her energy and blood sugar level.

Curvaceous **Dolly Parton** eats everything she ate when heavy, but much smaller portions of it. She still enjoys her favourite snack of all, Velveeta Cheese, but just a few bites.

Jane Seymour satisfies her sweet tooth with frozen fruit bars. She had no problem getting her 5´4˝ figure back after delivering twins.

Singer/actress **Vanessa Williams** won't touch caffeine or wheat. How did she come to this dietary conclusion? She consulted a psychic!

Friends star **Jennifer Aniston** used to weigh 30 pounds more than her now svelte 112 pounds. This 5´5˝ cutie stopped eating mayonnaise sandwiches and fried foods and discovered the health benefits of low-fat foods.

Suzanne Somers' weight problems caused her to lose acting roles. She credits a trial and error approach of combining certain foods in daily diet. She has also eliminated some foods that she labels "funky" that helped her to lose 20 pounds. These include potatoes, white flour, sugars, caffeine, and alcohol.

Talk show host **Leeza Gibbons** uses "skinny" sauces like a combination of Dijon mustard combined with yoghurt over baked potatoes. She eats dessert, but chooses fat-free angel food cake topped with fruit. Other snacks like popcorn, carrot sticks, and chocolate-covered raisins keep at her weight of 130. This 5´8˝ beauty also hikes and runs, and uses the treadmill and stair stepper a couple of times a week.

Actress **Melanie Griffith** is a busy mum, and can't always get to a health club. She keeps her 5´9˝, 118–20 pound figure by biking, swimming, walking, and running. She concentrates on eating right, and drinks bottled water and juices throughout the day. Melanie believes in supplementing her diet with vitamins and minerals. She changes them from time to time, depending on what her body is needing.

"Wonder Woman" **Lynda Carter** fits in exercise when she can, and absolutely insists that it be something enjoyable. Her favourites include skiing, hiking, running, and in-line skating. "That way it's not a chore," she says. Lynda stands 5´9˝ and keeps her weight at 130.

Turning 50 never looked better than it does on beautiful **Jaclyn Smith**. Her spectacular 5´7˝, 115-pound figure is the result of giving up cheese and cream sauces. She concentrates on meals that are low in fat, but still enjoys burgers. She is sure to include 45-minute power walks into her regime at least two or three times a week.

Who doesn't admire **Julia Roberts**' long streamlined body? Although she swears that she doesn't do anything "special" to maintain her 5´10˝, 120 pounds, during filming she is known for downing 8 glasses of water a day.

Cheryl Tiegs, Still Model Material After 50

How does **Cheryl Tiegs**, supermodel of the 60s and 70s, still maintain that fabulous body after passing that 50-year mark? Fitness is a constant in her life, and she stays on top of it on a daily basis. She claims to have kept a steady diet all her life.

Breakfast: it's something crunchy like Shredded Wheat or Grape-Nuts for fibre.
Lunch: the biggest meal of Cheryl's day, grilled meat, vegetables, and a salad

Dinner: fish, chicken, or meat with vegetables
Snacks: air-popped popcorn, occasional dessert

Exercise for Cheryl varies: aerobic conditioning, sit-ups, free weights, tennis, and hiking. The result? A weigh-in of 134 pounds every morning (she's 5´10˝). She watches her weight diligently.

A Big Problem Resolved!
Former Playboy Playmate of the Year **Anna Nicole Smith** blames her love of Southern-fried foods along with the death of her husband for ballooning her weight from 155 to 220 pounds. The 5´11˝ buxom beauty combined weight training and aerobic workouts to achieve her 60-pound weight loss to take off that gain.

Feeding Cravings
That's the secret behind *Friends* star **Courtney Cox**. She is known for nibbling on sweets all day long on the set. Admitting to a very strong sweet tooth, Courtney compensates by eating lightly at night. Running and power yoga are also a "must" in her daily activity to allow her to indulge in her munching.

Julia Louis-Dreyfus
The only woman brave enough to go up against the *Seinfield* crew gained 65 pounds during her last pregnancy. Standing at a petite 5´3˝, she worked fervently to get back into shape. She limits red meats and concentrates on fish, pasta, fruit, and vegetables. Julia has worked with both a nutritionist and a personal trainer to resolve her post-pregnancy weight gains.

Listening to Her Body

It's hard to believe that gorgeous actress/comedienne **Lisa Kudrow** eats whatever she wants and yet stays a curvy 5´7˝ and 123 pounds. Her secret is listening to her body, and differentiating between cravings, physical hunger, and body satisfaction. Lisa claims that there is an inner voice that tells her when she's had enough to eat. Although there are no foods that she can't or won't eat, she limits herself to certain favourite sweets.

Relaxing about Food

Whenever former *Melrose Place* actress **Josie Bissett** ate biscuits, she would then figure out just how she could exercise it off. Stopping the obsession has given her peace of mind and greatly reduced her stress level.

Moderate Lifestyle Leads to Moderate Eating

The funny thing about model **Frederique** (best known for her layouts in *Victoria's Secret* catalogues) is that her diet is fairly normal. Born in the Netherlands, she was brought up in a culture where dieting is not part of the culture. She has brought with her the idea that it IS possible to eat one slice of cheese and an occasional piece of chocolate. Another crazy idea she's brought over from her country? She eats when she gets hungry.

How the Stars Handle Weight Gains

Actress **Salma Hayek** says that when she gains a few pounds she stops eating dinner for a few days. Her ideal weight is a remarkable 106 pounds.

Growing up in an Italian family gave **Mira Sorvino** a lifelong love of pasta, red wine and pizza. Mira has said that food is like sex: "When it's great it's amazing, and when it's OK it's still pretty good." When she needs to drop a few pounds, as she did to play a bulimic in *Beautiful Girls*, she sticks to salad, grilled chicken, and sushi.

Sharon Lawrence reportedly went on a crash diet to do her now famous nude scene in *NYPD Blue*. She survived on water and clear soup alone for several days before the shooting.

Being petite makes it even more difficult for **Toni Braxton** to keep those remarkable curves. Her figure has been the topic of great admiration. She loves to show off those curves with body-revealing evening gowns. She got that way by practising incredible restraint in the foods she selected. Hardest for her was eliminating beer and nuts (together they are deadly!).

A healthy lifestyle is the hallmark of longtime model **Christie Brinkley's** all-American body. This fish-eating vegetarian keeps junk food out of the house to ensure that when weight gains occur, snacking is done on sweet potatoes and not chocolate bars. When she needs to lose weight quickly, she slims down on a liquid diet of fruit and vegetable juices, mixed with acidophilus.

When **Jamie Lee Curtis**, aka The Body, had to lose five pounds for her role in *True Lies*, she cut all fat from her diet and ate nothing but vegetables.

> **Curvy Kate Winslet** has been raked with public criticism ranging from fashion designers to showbiz news groups on the Internet. Kate has battled her weight since her teenage years, and was called "Blubber" by her fellow classmates. She was able to diet down to a size ten for her role in *Titanic* by eating sensibly rather than crash dieting.

Kirstie Alley is subject to continual criticism of her weight fluctuations. Knowing that she has to stay competitive in the very visible acting world, she sometimes resorts to drinking only herbal teas for a couple of days.

Marilu Henner went from 160 pounds to 121 (she's 5´7˝) by eliminating all dairy products from her diet. She also eliminated all caffeine and refined sugars.

Statuesque *3rd Rock From the Sun* star **Kristen Johnsen** drops weight by cutting out desserts, between meal snacks, and butter on her bread. She substitutes lemon juice for salad dressing.

The Power of Protein

Although actress and former model **Cameron Diaz** has a fast metabolism, it may be her unusual way of starting her day that helps her keep her 5´9˝, 120-pound perfect shape. Cameron eats a big serving of chicken! She claims it provides her with a quick energy start.

Actress **Lisa Rinna** chooses a chocolate protein shake for breakfast, blended with a banana. When she wants to drop a few pounds, Lisa cuts back on the amount of carbohydrates she's eating, and also adds more protein to her diet.

Figure skater **Peggy Fleming** stays low on carbohydrates and high on protein. Just a half-cup of rice for dinner and a slice of toast for breakfast for this beautiful 50-year-old gold medallist.

Sensible Body Talk

Actress and former model **Andie McDowell** is a very healthy 5´8˝ and weighs in at 125 to 130 pounds. This proponent of a macrobiotic diet is a big opponent of the waif look of the model industry and the unhealthy lifestyle sometimes used to attain the image. You won't find her working out in a gym, but more likely riding horses on her family's ranch in Montana.

Revelations of Emotional Eating

Singer **Janet Jackson** explained in *Ebony* that food had become her favorite anaesthetic. "I escaped through eating," she confesses. "Certain things may happen, and you dismiss them instead of stopping and saying, 'Why am I feeling this way? Why am I acting out in this way?'"

Defying Age

Sophia Loren is the doyen of discipline. For years she has talked about her love of pasta, but before you start digging in, listen to what she doesn't eat. Sophia rarely eats meat, and drinks lots of water. You won't find her eating potato chips, smoking cigarettes, or drinking an alcoholic beverage. Cheese, fruit and vegetables make up the rest of her daily meals.

How does "Supreme" diva **Diana Ross** stay in shape? She does her own housework. "Cleaning is a tremendous stress reliever and it keeps my body taut," says Diana. Any 25-year-old would have a hard time competing with this 5´4˝, 100-pound 53-year-old.

Yoga plays a major role in the wonderful condition **Raquel Welch** is in at 57. She practises some form of it every day. A big protein eater (turkey, veal, fish, some red meat), other snacks include rice cakes and fresh fruit.

> "The body is a machine. You train it to do what you want it to do."
> Tina Turner

Stirring honey into her coffee or tea helps **Ann-Margret** stay away from sweets. This motorcycle-driving actress and singer watches her diet by avoiding fizzy drinks, sweets, and peanuts. She also reportedly went on a watermelon diet for two weeks to drop 20 pounds. She ate watermelon for breakfast and lunch along with lots of water. At dinner, she would eat a low-fat, nourishing meal.

No snacks for former "Mamas and Papas" singer and *Knots Landing* actress **Michelle Phillips**. This 54-year-old owes her 5´7˝, 120-pound figure to fresh fruit and vegetables, supplemented by daily vitamins.

Faye Dunaway claims she is in better condition today at 56 than at any other time in her life. There is no white flour in her diet, just lots of salads, grilled fish, and vegetables, and seven-grain breads.

You can count **Goldie Hawn** as one of the lovely over-50 actresses who occasionally fasts on juice to detoxify and keep her in shape.

Barbara Eden of *I Dream of Jeannie* fame chooses lunch as her biggest meal of the day, because her body will have at least 10 hours to digest it.

Water and yoga have allowed **Ali McGraw** to remain 59 years young. She credits water with keeping her blood flowing, her muscles pumping, and her hair and skin healthy.

Catwoman **Eartha Kitt** likes to keep her weight at about 122. She's a mere 5´3˝, so if she finds herself five pounds over her ideal she increases her activity level by cleaning her house, and taking a two-mile walk.

Dynasty's **Linda Evans**, now 55, has been able to lose 25 pounds thanks to 30 minutes of daily aerobics. She has so fervently embraced the exercise world that she has recently opened a chain of her own fitness centres. She is now able to keep her 5´8˝ frame at about 136 pounds.

Chapter Six

Diet Emergencies

Crash Diets Can Work!

A crash diet isn't always a bad thing, and many times it really works! Emergency diets have the ability to inspire the dieter by the quick results seen over just a few days. Although the weight loss is mostly water, some fat is also lost. The other benefits are a flatter stomach, a sense of well being, and reduced bulges around the hips and thighs. Here are some of the most successful "quick start" diets.

The One-Day Juice Fast

This diet is probably the most popular "one day only" diet (besides fasting) that has been used to drop about two to three pounds in one day without using any supplements. Fresh juices have great nutritional value, and contain important enzymes, minerals, and vitamins. They cleanse your system, and make you feel like you could conquer the world!

7 a.m.: A cup of hot water with the juice of one lemon or one teaspoon of reconstituted lemon juice.

8 a.m.: Apple-carrot juice consisting of 4 unpeeled carrots and two unpeeled, cored apples.

10 a.m.: A glass of water or a cup of herbal tea.

12 p.m.: A large glass of grapefruit juice and a large glass of iced water.

2 p.m.: A glass of water and a cup of herbal tea.

4 p.m.: A glass of pineapple juice and a glass of iced water.

6 p.m.: Herbal tea and a glass of water.

8 p.m.: Pineapple or grapefruit juice with a glass of iced water.

10 p.m.: A cup of hot water with the juice of one lemon or one teaspoon of reconstituted lemon.

If you find that you have a difficult time getting to sleep after a day of this juice diet, try adding a few special herbs to your bath. Visit your local health food store, where you'll find oils to help you relax. Look for essences of rose, sandalwood, and lavender. To enjoy wonderfully natural aromatherapy, just cut up a lemon or orange and throw it in. These are the basis of citric cleaners, and will make your bathtub shine! Herbal tea bags also create a relaxing bath treatment. Especially soothing are cloves, peppermint, and chamomile.

The Cabbage Diet

This diet has been passed around forever. It's been called the Model's Diet, the Stewardess Diet, even the Dolly Parton Diet. I don't really know whose diet it is, but lots of people have had tremendous success with it.

Diet Soup Recipe
2 to 3 cubes of bouillon
1 package onion soup mix
3 onions
1 to 2 head of cabbage
2 to 3 pounds of tomatoes
1 carrot
1 pepper
Seasonings to taste

Blanch tomatoes in boiling water for one minute. Plunge into cold water, remove skins, and set aside. Dissolve soup mix and bouillon in 3 quarts of water. Chop and then add cabbage, onion, carrot, pepper, and spices. Add tomatoes. Bring to a boil and cook for 30 to 40 minutes. Makes enough soup for 2 days.

Eat all the Diet Soup you want for 7 days along with the following:

1st day: fruits only

2nd day: vegetables only

3rd day: fruits and vegetables

4th day: 8 bananas and nonfat milk

5th day: 6 ounces lean poultry or fish and plain rice

6th day: same as 5th day

7th day: vegetables and rice

"I've tried this diet along with everyone at my office, and it does work. The only problem is the weight comes off so fast that it's very easy to gain it back when you stop the diet. All my friends agree that it's a great way to get started on a new healthy lifestyle. On the day that calls for banana and milk, I make a milkshake. I also like to use a lot of spices on my fish, poultry, and vegetables."

Markie, age 27, 38 pounds lost

The Grapefruit Diet

This is a diet that doesn't require a lot of planning or thought. You don't need to count calories or make major food decisions. The plus side to this diet is that grapefruit contains so much fibre and water, it fills you up quickly. The downside is that it's too restrictive to be healthy for more than a couple of days.

Breakfast: Half a grapefruit with coffee or tea.
Lunch: Two eggs, lettuce and tomato salad spritzed with lemon

and vinegar, a slice of toast, half a grapefruit, and coffee or tea.
Dinner: Fish or chicken, half a grapefruit, cucumbers or tomatoes, and coffee or tea.

The High-Protein Diet

We saw the start of this craze with the late Dr Stillman's Scarsdale Diet. It's still very much alive, and has been incorporated into many diets today. *The Zone*, *Protein Power*, and *Dr Atkins' Diet Revolution* all are based on the protein theory   that too many carbohydrates prevent the body from burning fat. Typically the protein diet goes like this:

Breakfast: Eggs and bacon (unrestricted amounts), but no toast or juice allowed.
Lunch: Small salad and cheeseburger (no bun).
Dinner: Steak or fried chicken and a salad with blue-cheese dressing.

The Liquid Diet

This is certainly one of the most convenient diets around today. Slimfast, Nestle Sweet Success, etc. allow you to simply open a can, get a glass, and add milk. These shakes are nutritionally balanced and typically contain about 20 vitamins and minerals. The rule is to eliminate two meals a day with the shake, and eat a third meal consisting of no more than 500 to 600 calories. Each drink will contain about 200 calories and only 1 to 3 grams of fat. The problem that dieters face with this plan is that the oral satiety level is not fulfilled.

"I felt deprived on these 'milkshakes'. I was desperate to chew, and found myself sticking an average of 15 to 20 pieces of gum in my mouth daily. Although I initially lost a lot of weight, it gradually came back when I stopped using the shakes. I did like the convenience, and even now will bring one to the office in case I can't get out."

Penny, age 45, 22 pounds lost

The Mini Meal Diet

Eating food only three times a day, at breakfast, lunch, and dinner, is too restricting for many dieters. Being able to "graze" throughout the day, especially when cutting drastically back on calories, boosts the success rate radically. This plan allows for eating six times a day, and still will yield an average weight loss of five to six pounds in three days. It's easy to follow and really quite painless!

Menu One

Breakfast
1 cup Frosted Shredded Wheat with skimmed milk
Coffee or tea

Snack
½ cup cubed cantaloupe or one apple

Lunch
4 ounces sliced turkey breast on wholegrain bread with 1 teaspoon mustard
Mixed green salad
Coffee, tea, or diet beverage

Snack
1 cup skimmed milk
1 chocolate chip cookie

Dinner
3 ounces broiled chicken or fish (any)
1 cup cooked spinach
Coffee, tea, or iced water

Snack
6 ounces low-fat yoghurt

Menu Two

Breakfast
½ cup strawberries
6 ounces low-fat yoghurt
Coffee or tea

Snack
½ cup baby carrots
6 pretzels

Lunch
1 cup canned vegetable soup
4 saltine crackers
Coffee, tea, or diet beverage

Snack
1 apple

Dinner
3 ounces sirloin steak
1 cup sliced green beans
Coffee, tea, or iced water

Snack
½ cup low-fat frozen yoghurt

This diet works quickly and efficiently because you know that you'll be eating again in just two hours. Those of us who are parents know that when our children are young, it's important to bring along snacks if we plan to be away from home for a long period of time. Yet, we never anticipate our own hunger, which can lead to that stop at the vending machine, fast food drive-in, and the downfall of our best intentions of the morning. Snacking is important as an energy restorative as well as for staving off hunger pains.

Celebrity Crash Plans

Donna Karan
When designer Donna Karan wants to lose a few pounds quickly, she turns to her favourite detoxifying juice. In a food processor, blend the following ingredients: 1/4 wedge of cabbage, 1 red apple, 6 sprigs parsley, 3 carrots, 3 stalks celery.

Melanie Griffith
"I eat nothing but fruit in the mornings when I'm trying to lose weight."

Joan Collins
When actress Joan Collins needs to lose weight quickly in order to flatten her tummy into a slinky *Dynasty*-type gown, she'll stop eating for an entire day. Sometimes all it takes is to eliminate one dinner.

Damage Control
Celebrities who make their living from the way they look immediately take care of any small weight gains. They don't let the problem run away from them. Their contracts, in fact their very fortunes, depend on it. It's a habit everyone should adopt into their lives.

General Emergency Measures

Stay Away from Sodium

Hide the salt shaker for a few days to shed those pounds quickly. Also stay away from canned soups, salty snacks, and processed foods.

Eat More Protein

Choose protein wisely and stay away from nuts and beans. Go for lean meats, poultry, fish and egg whites.

Eat Less Carbohydrates

Limit your carbs to two a day and you'll find that the pounds will come off quickly. Your best choices are cereal (go for at least five grams of fibre), potatoes and grain-based breads.

Avoid Carbonated Beverages

Even low-calorie drinks can give you a false bloated appearance.

Limit Added Fat

Try not to consume more than one tablespoon of salad dressing, butter, or other oil a day.

Eat Fat-Free Fruits

The fruits you select make a big difference in the weight-loss game. Go for apples, pears, bananas, grapefruit, blueberries and oranges.

Load Up on Fat-Free Vegetables

You can eat to your heart's content the following vegetables: green beans, broccoli, carrots, spinach, celery, mushrooms, tomatoes, and Romaine lettuce. Use these vegetables to refuel your body between meals, or whenever you get ravenous.

Drink Lots of Water

Don't worry, you are not going to add bloat by downing lots of water. On the contrary, the more you drink, the more easily your body will excrete it. When not enough water is absorbed into the body, a survival measure goes into gear, and the body holds on to what it has. Don't forget to add lots of ice to rev up the metabolism. Water will also increase elimination.

The Spa 3-Day Diet

Try this diet on a relaxing weekend. It's sure to bring a satisfying 5- to 6-pound weight loss. Try to incorporate it into a "makeover" time for you. Wear your workout clothes and take a hike around your neighbourhood. Test out those homemade masks and hair treatments you've been anxious to try, but felt too busy.

Day One

Breakfast
2 frozen low-fat waffles topped with 1/2 cup blueberries and a teaspoon of low-fat topping
Coffee or tea

Lunch
1 cup mixed greens with 1 ounce water-packed tuna and 2 tablespoons low-fat dressing or mayonnaise
Alfalfa sprouts and red peppers to taste
1 slice protein or wholegrain bread
Diet beverage

Dinner

3 ounces chicken breast coated with 1 tablespoon each Dijon mustard, honey, and apple-cider vinegar
Sprinkle with basil and broil
2 cups mixed greens topped with 2 tablespoons low-fat dressing
Coffee or tea

Day Two

Breakfast

½ grapefruit
1 slice pita bread toasted with 1 ounce Swiss or muenster cheese
Coffee or tea

Lunch

Mix ¼ cup grapes, pineapple slices, kiwi, and strawberries with 1 cup yoghurt. Sprinkle with 2 teaspoons wheatgerm.
Diet beverage, coffee or tea

Dinner

1 cup pasta of choice topped with ½ cup marinara sauce and 1 teaspoon parmesan cheese
1 cup steamed zucchini
2 cups mixed greens tossed with 2 tablespoons low-fat dressing
Coffee or tea

Day Three

Breakfast

1 slice raisin bread broiled with 1 tablespoon low-fat cottage cheese topped with cinnamon
½ cup fruit
Coffee or tea

Lunch

1 slice pita bread broiled with 1 ounce mozzarella cheese, sliced

tomatoes, and your choice of mushrooms, broccoli, and onions
2 cups mixed greens with 2 tablespoons low-fat dressing
Diet beverage

Dinner
3 ounces white fish broiled with 1 teaspoon sesame oil and
sesame seeds, topped with ginger
½ cup wild rice
1 cup broccoli
Coffee, tea or diet beverage

Each day choose from two of the following snacks:
1 cup cubed cantaloupe
½ cup banana blended with ½ cup skimmed milk, 1 teaspoon
vanilla, and 4 ice cubes
½ cup skimmed milk and 1 low-fat biscuit

Two-Day Pasta Diet
Here's good news for pasta lovers. There's a fun diet going
around that allows for your favourite food plus a 3- to 4-pound
quick weight loss. Sound impossible? Try it, and you'll find it
one of the easiest diets you've been on in a long time.

Day One

Breakfast
4 scrambled egg whites and ¼ cup mushrooms
1 slice low calorie bread
Coffee or tea

Lunch
1 cup cold pasta mixed with 2 ounces tuna and 1 tablespoon
low-fat dressing
1 teaspoon grated cheese
Diet beverage

Dinner

1 ½ cup spaghetti topped with ½ cup tomato sauce and 1 ounce browned meat

1 teaspoon grated cheese

Coffee, tea or iced water

Day Two

Breakfast

½ cup low-fat cottage cheese with ½ cup pineapple

1 slice low-calorie bread

Coffee or tea

Lunch

1 cup egg noodles mixed with 1 ounce chopped chicken or turkey, 1 ounce melted part-skimmed mozzarella cheese, and 1 cup cooked spinach

Diet beverage

Dinner

1 ½ cups macaroni mixed with 2 ounces low-fat melted cheddar cheese.

Mixed green salad with 1 tablespoon salad dressing blended with 1 tablespoon balsamic vinegar

Coffee, tea, or iced water

Chapter Seven

Supplements

Supplements for Weight Loss

You've heard it a million times. The safest and most effective way to lose weight is to eat less. If it were that easy, everyone would be losing all kinds of weight. Well, the good news is that there are supplements and herbs that really do work to provide that extra edge.

Chitosan

This natural fibre is found in lobster shells and acts like a fat magnet when taken 15 minutes before eating. Since it is non-digestible and binds with dietary fat, it quickly passes out of the body along with fat from the meal you've just eaten, report researchers. A study revealed that people taking Chitosan lost an average of eight per cent of their body weight. The effect is reportedly enhanced when taken with orange or lemon juice before a meal.

Chromium Picolinate

Scientists have discovered that people who lack chromium in their bodies carry extra weight. The supplements chromium picolinate and chromium polynicotate have been around for a few years. Chromium is an essential dietary nutrient which plays an important role in processing fat and carbohydrates. Many users report that it cuts sweet cravings, too. You could use this supplement if your diet lacks chromium-rich foods. These foods include mushrooms, apples, broccoli and cheese. The recommended daily allowance is anywhere from 50 to 200 micrograms. Supplements are usually sold in 200 micrograms, or mixed with other products in varying amounts. This product is readily available in drugstores, health food stores, supermarkets and general merchandisers.

CLA

Conjugated Linoleic Acid (CLA) is a fatty acid marketed under the name Tonalin. Its purpose is to reduce fat by inhibiting the body's ability to store fats. CLA also increases muscle tone, improves food efficiency, and contains antioxidant properties.

Coenzyme Q10

Useful for obesity, coronary heart disease, lack of energy, and high cholesterol levels. Studies have found that some overweight people have low levels of Coenzyme Q10 (CoQ10) and by supplementing it they can help control their body weight. Recommended dose is for up to 90 milligrams of CoQ10 without side effects. Anyone with heart disease should first check with their doctor.

Creatine

This noncaloric enzyme can safely create better muscle tone and increase endurance for longer workouts. Creatine works by helping the body retain water in the muscle tissue, which helps to heal the muscle more efficiently without bloating the body. Recommended dosage is 10 to 20 grams a day for the first week, then 5 grams a day. Creatine monohydrate is available in capsules, bars, and shakes.

Garcinia Cambogia

Garcinia cambogia is a yellow fruit from Southeast Asia. Used in cooking, the garcinia extract is added to make meals more filling. Said to aid digestion, it contains hydroxyl citric aid, which is similar to the citric acid in citrus fruits.

Research conducted in the 1970s at Brandeis University, and later by Hoffman-LaRoche (the pharmaceutical company), showed that rats fed hydroxyl citrate shed 25 per cent of their body fat in 22 days. The rats lost body fat partly because hydroxyl citric acid inhibits an enzyme that converts surplus carbohydrate calories into fat.

Available in pill form and in bars at health food stores, garcinia cambogia has taken the natural weight loss industry by storm. It controls the appetite in a natural, safe way, and has no known side effects. It is unlike any of the chemicals sold as diet pills.

Garcinia cambogia is a supplement that is most effective taken 30 to 60 minutes before meals. Take it with a glass of water or with a piece of fruit. Taking it with a bowl of soup also seems to help.

Glutamine

This amino acid promotes uptake of nutrients to build muscle tissue.

HMB

The latest fat-burning and muscle-building supplement to impress experts is beta-hydroxy-methylbutyrate (HMB). Studies showed that taking 3 grams of this protein substance daily caused athletes to gain 63 per cent more muscle size and strength and lose twice as much fat as those exercisers who didn't take it.

L-Carnitine

This supplement is reported to accelerate the benefits of chromium. Leading fitness buffs and die-hard weight watchers take the two together. It is sold both as a separate unit, and in combination with other supplements. L-Carnitine is an amino acid which may be in short supply in many diets. The recommended dosage for this supplement is from 250 to 500 milligrams daily.

Meridia

This is a prescription drug that is meant to be safer than its predecessors, fen-phen and Redux. It will be prescribed only for people with a body mass index of 30 or above. Owing to the history of problems with other prescription weight-loss products, it would be well advised to check that your physician has been properly informed about Meridia.

Orlistat

A new prescription diet drug that works directly on the intestine. It is part of a group of drugs called "lipase inhibitors". Lipase is an enzyme in the intestine that breaks down fat. This drug works on that enzyme to prevent the absorption of fat by about 30 per cent.

Phen Cal-106

A combination of amino acids that works against the major causes of weight-gain, cravings, and bingeing. Originally developed to deal with substance abuse, the amino acids feed the brain. The brain becomes satisfied. You can also purchase the four amino acids in this product separately at your local health food store. They are: phenylalanine, glutamine, tyrosine, and tryptophan.

Pregnenolone

A hormone that is produced naturally in our bodies that decreases after the age of 35. Not only does it contain anti-ageing benefits, but it makes it easier for people to lose weight and improve muscle. It also improves skin tone. Recommended dosage is 10 milligrams two or three times a week.

Pyruvate

Found in red apples, and now available in capsule form, this natural substance has almost 30 years of research to back up its claims and safety features. Use it to help burn fats and carbohydrates more efficiently.

Vanadyl Sulfate

This nutrient helps build lean muscle tissue by increasing amino acid uptake.

A Word about Appetite Suppressants

For those of you who use over-the-counter diet aids to suppress your appetite be aware of the following:

Purchase the cheapest brand available. They all contain the same basic ingredients.

Don't take more than the recommended dosage. There have been reports of strokes and deaths related to the misuse of these products. It is always recommended that you check with your doctor before taking them.

Herbs That Help Shed Pounds

There are herbs you can add to your diet as supplements, teas, and foods that will help your weight-loss programme go smoothly. Some can even be sprinkled into your bath.

Sibutramine

A new prescription-only appetite suppressant that works by maintaining high levels of serotonin, the blood chemical that triggers fullness. Those taking it experience fewer cravings and eat less. The most exciting results of extensive studies is that it enabled two out of three people to lose 5 to 10 per cent of their body fat safely and without additional dieting or exercising.

Alfalfa
Aids digestion and acts as a diuretic. It belongs to the special vegetable family of nitrogen-fixing legumes.

Aloe Powder
Causes temporary water-weight reduction because of its strong laxative effects.

Aloe Vera
Helps to maintain regularity, among its other benefits.

Bladder Wrack
Improves thyroid function and is a bulk laxative.

Burdock
Improves fat metabolism and acts as a diuretic.

Capsicum
This will produce heat to rev up the metabolism and burn fat.

Cardamom
Improves circulation and digestion. A thermogenic herb.

Cayenne
Improves circulation and digestion. Has thermogenic effects.

Chickweed
Long reported as a weight loss tool by herbalists, but not widely tested scientifically.

Cinnamon
Creates a thermogenic burn.

Dandelion Root
Aids fat metabolism by affecting the liver.

Ephedra (Ma Huang)
Without a doubt the most controversial herb on the market today. Some have called it "legalized speed". It stimulates the nervous system, suppressing appetite. It also allegedly speeds metabolism. The side effects are dizziness, jitters, insomnia, and heart palpitations. Abusing the dosage has led to stroke, heart attack, and seizures.

Fennel
A diuretic that reduces hunger and improves energy.

Flax Seed
A bulk laxative that helps curb hunger. Flax swells in the stomach and intestines to promote a sense of fullness.

Garcinia Cambogia
Aids fat metabolism and reduces hunger.

Green Tea
Aids fat metabolism and increases energy.

> ## Ch'i-111
>
> This all-natural herbal formulation (pronounced Chi-3) blends 12 herbs from China, India, and the Amazon rain forest with Western nutrients. Its purpose is to help create thermogenesis in the body. This will speed up the body's removal of fat from the adipose tissue (white fat). It also acts as an appetite suppressant. Follow the recommended dosage on the product's label.

Guarana

Helps to reduce hunger and has a laxative effect. It contains caffeine, and is reported to speed metabolism and burn fat.

Gymnema Tea

Is your problem a sweet tooth? Gymnema tea coats your tongue, tricking it into finding real sugar bland. The effect lasts for two to three hours. Dieters report that it takes away their desire for doughnuts, cakes, biscuits, etc.

Hawthorn

Reduces blood fat and improves circulation.

Kava

This distant cousin to black pepper contains ingredients that produce physical and mental relaxation. Especially useful for stress-related eating.

Kelp

This is a sea plant that is available in capsule form. It helps thyroid function, which regulates the metabolism.

Kola Nut
A stimulant that decreases appetite and aids in the metabolism of fat.

Papaya
Aids digestion.

Parsley
A diuretic and nutritional aid.

Phyllium
Helps to curb hunger and allow the elimination of wastes from the body.

Senna
An all-natural laxative. It is found in weight-loss teas to stimulate the colon. To be used occasionally. Just like any other laxative, it can become habit forming.

Spirulina
Also known as blue-green algae, spirulina contains a natural appetite suppressant. It is a rich source of phenylalanine, a naturally occurring substance that helps create a feeling of fullness after eating.

Stevia
A little-known South American herb called Stevia rebaudiana-bertoni has not one caloric, yet is up to 300 times sweeter than sugar. Use it in its powder form to sweeten beverages. It's a natural alternative to aspartame and saccharin.

Valerian Root
If stress sends you right to the refrigerator, this natural tranquiliser will stop you from pigging out.

Vinegar

Ancient healers have used vinegar for thousands of years. Take two teaspoons of vinegar mixed with a glass of water at each meal. The vinegar will help your body to burn fat, rather than store it. Use any vinegar that appeals to you. Apple cider vinegar is a delicious flavour to try. Vinegar is a natural storehouse of vitamins and minerals. Experiment and come up with the tastes that you've never before experienced.

Aspirin for Weight Loss

An aspirin a day will burn away fat! The key is thermogenesis, the chemical process by which your body generates heat and speeds up your natural metabolism. Aspirin revs up the metabolism, making it run faster, burn hotter, and vaporise fat effortlessly. Less fat in the body can also unclog arteries and slash your risk of heart attack and stroke by 50 per cent. Of course, you should check with your doctor.

Vitamins and Supplements for Health and Well Being

You are cutting down on calories, but you do not want to cut back on nutrients. In most weight-loss programmes, the requisite vitamins are not being consumed. Here are some of the supplements used to balance out a reduced-calorie diet.

Bee Pollen

The buzz on bee pollen is that it gives you an extra energy lift. Be sure to take small doses of it in the beginning. Some users have found that they are allergic to it. It's known as the "alternative to coffee" by holistic groups.

Cat's Claw

Known as the Peruvian wonder herb, cat's claw is the newest

herb to come out of the ancient rain forest of the Amazon. A natural antioxidant, one of the major benefits is that it is anti-edemic (takes down swelling). Use it for swollen ankles, bloating, and PMS.

Dang Gui
Also known as dong quai and tang kuei, this is one of the most versatile herbs available today. From the name, it is obvious that its origins are in Chinese medicine. It has been used to treat menstrual abnormalities (cramps, PMS) and menopausal symptoms. It is also useful in treating respiratory problems, and even gas.

Echinacea
Rich in polysaccharides, echinacea helps to activate the immune cells. It naturally inhibits inflammation. Widely used in Europe, take it only when you feel an illness coming on. It has no cumulative effects.

Evening Primrose Oil
Particularly popular in England, it benefits the skin and hair, and is said to aid in hair restoration.

Folic Acid
Helps the immune system and blood building. Plays a role in promoting DNA and RNA to make new cells.

Garlic
Take the deodorised tablets for benefits in lowering high blood pressure.

Ginger
It prevents motion sickness and relieves nausea. Ginger is also reported to prevent and heal ulcers.

Ginkgo Biloba

Good circulation is vital to supplying a healthy brain with the food and oxygen it needs. The ginkgo tree, derived from the oldest living tree, has many benefits. It increases alertness, improves memory, and lowers cholesterol levels. But more importantly (to our looks), there's evidence that ginkgo may be the most potent anti-ager ever! The only problem I have come across if that there's no agreed-upon standard for the right amount to take. About 40 milligrams seems to be the recommended dosage from most sources I have solicited.

St. John's Wort

Known as the natural alternative to Prozac, it works to increase the production of the brain chemical serotonin, boosting mood and curbing overeating associated with depression. It's often used in combination with ephedra to battle weight problems, especially eating disorders and binge eating.

Ginseng

This popular supplement has many health and longevity benefits. It improves energy levels and enhances mental alertness. It has immune-strengthening benefits and is able to lower cholesterol levels. Ginseng is reported to decrease the chance of heart disease and increase good cholesterol levels.

Grape Seeds

Antioxidants in grape seeds protect the thin walls of blood vessels from losing their strength. Beauties use it to prevent and correct the appearance of spider veins.

Grapefruit Seed Extract
Made from the seeds and pulp of grapefruits, grapefruit seed extract is receiving praise from both holistic and mainstream medical researchers. Its properties boost the immune system. It is also proclaimed to be an alternative to antibiotics. It is reported to fight bacteria, viruses, and parasites, which is why it is most used for flus, colds, sore throats, and even yeast infections.

Iron
A trace mineral that carries oxygen to cells to produce energy, iron helps the immune system operate at peak efficiency.

Kombucha Mushroom
This health craze is a living organism of bacteria and yeast, and has been used for centuries in China and Russia. One of its key ingredients is said to be glucuronic acid, a detoxifying agent. Devotees say kombucha tea improves well-being and energy
levels. It's sold in many forms, and many beauties are making teas out of it, grow it — everything but wear it. I have heard some negatives about its safety, so do be careful. Some health professionals are concerned about the safety of the brew. If you would like to give it a try, I'd go with the tablet form, available at drugstores and vitamin outlets.

Lavender Oil
Use it in drop form in the bath, to alleviate stress, and to ease headache pain.

Licorice Root
Long used in Germany, this helps with vitamin absorption and the prevention of ulcers.

Melatonin

A supplement that, in addition to being the ultimate sleeping pill, eliminates jet lag, and improves mood. It is also reported to enhance the immune system, treat a variety of diseases, and even prolong life. The biggest claims that have been reported (but as of yet unproven) are that it can reverse the ageing process, fight cancers, and even prevent pregnancy. Most doctors, scientists, and nutritionists agree that from one to three milligrams is the recommended dosage.

Pycnogenol

A compound form of the French maritime pine, this is a most powerful antioxidant that acts in a similar way to vitamin E, but with fifty times the strength. It boasts twenty times the strength of vitamin C. Use it to protect cell membranes from sun damage.

Beta Carotene

This vitamin A precursor protects lipids in cell membranes and between skin cells from free radical attack. In everyday language, beta carotene makes the skin stay moist, supple, and youthful.

Royal Jelly

This is one of the most enduringly popular food supplements. Swathed in the mysteries of ancient China and the East where it was first discovered, royal jelly, in its raw state, is a unique high-protein food. It is produced by bees and fed to their offspring. Used by us as a food supplement, it is available in both capsule and liquid forms. Loyal followers prefer the liquid because it can be more easily absorbed into the system. Also use it to boost your energy levels.

Seaweed

What you used to avoid at the beach has many health benefits. It's sold in both dried form and tablets. You can reconstitute it and add it to your salads and soups as many models do. If seaweed doesn't exactly tempt your taste buds, go for the tablets. The most popular tablets are Dulse and Kelp. Take it for the rehydrating benefits. Seaweed is also able to boost a sluggish thyroid.

Selenium

Take this vitamin to enhance the effects of vitamin E. Selenium has a close metabolic interrelationship with vitamin E, and will aid in body growth.

Vitamin A

Take this supplement to regulate skin hydration, aid eyesight, and repair skin and nails.

Vitamin B

This important vitamin keeps skin smooth, promotes hair and nail growth, and improves circulation.

Vitamin B-1 (Thiamine)

Stabilises appetite, stimulates growth, and helps metabolism.

Vitamin C

Available in several forms, it is quickly becoming the darling of the cosmetics industry. Vitamin C prolongs the life of vitamin E, protects immune cells in the skin to fight off cancer and other sun-related diseases. It also has been proven to fade age spots and other pigment irregularities. Of course, vitamin C also fends off colds.

Vitamin D

Promotes absorption of calcium and phosphorus and helps deposit these minerals in bones and teeth.

Vitamin E

Known as the skin vitamin, it has properties to heal scar tissue and neutralise damaging free radicals.

Wheat Grass Juice

Here's yet another purported natural energy enhancer. It is also used in homeopathic healing of some diseases.

Of course, you should try to get some of these nutrients in a multivitamin so that you're not spending half your day downing vitamins. That said, you'll become aware of what your body requires. Also note that vitamins should be taken with meals to help your body absorb them.

Chapter Eight

Exercise

Getting Started

You need to exercise. You'll lose weight faster and more efficiently if you do. Of course, exercise is also good for your health. The good news is that you don't need as much of it as the media has hyped. You simply need to start moving that body of yours. I'm sure you agree that we can easily become exhausted physically and mentally by some of the extremes celebrities and trainers go to on a daily basis to stay in shape. Who has the time or for that matter who cares to spend two or three hours in a gym every day?

Exercising Doesn't Require a Lot of "Stuff"
A lot of dieters fail to incorporate an exercise programme into their dieting plans because they think they can't afford the pricey equipment. You can certainly get a good workout with lots of equipment or by joining a gym, but it's truly not necessary. The successful dieters I interviewed for this book didn't credit their stair stepper or treadmill with being their key to long-term accomplishment.

Exercise Can Boost Creativity and Imagination
According to the *British Journal of Sports Medicine*, men and women aged 19 to 59 scored better on creativity tests after a

low- or high-impact workout. Studies also proved that mood was increased by 25 per cent after exercise.

You Just Have to Move

Do something you enjoy for 30 minutes a day. Hey, it might just be gardening or house cleaning. Walking to the library to find that perfect book or video is a good motivator as well. If you combine these 30 minutes with a low-calorie diet, the pounds will fall off, and that will become daily gratification.

Consult Your Doctor

Although your physician may very likely jump for joy when you mention it, it's a good idea to get checked out before beginning anything strenuous.

It Doesn't Matter the Time You Choose

According to several studies, including major research from Kansas State University, the number of calories burned will be roughly the same no matter when you work out. This was also the case with my own interviewees. The difference is that two-thirds of the calories burned by early morning exercise comes from fat deposits. It's cut to one-half if exercise is done in the afternoon or evening. Quite simply, though, the best time to exercise is when you're most likely to do it.

Make an Appointment with Yourself

This is your time just for you. If you can't find 30 minutes in your day, break it up into two 15-minute blocks. Imagine your body to be a piece of clay. You are the sculptor, and you know just how you want your arms, hips, and thighs to be sculpted. You'll be amazed at the strong, firm results.

Find a Friend

The right friend can make all the difference in the success of an exercise programme. Is there someone who's commiserated with you on their own weight problem? Do you know anyone who tends to be naturally competitive? Perhaps there's someone in your family who's been after you to lose weight? Knowing you have someone else who's cheering you on, or even that one person you know you have to answer to, is the concept that makes most diet clubs so successful. Even better, if you can get that person to engage in that exercise with you, you are going to stick with it.

Maybe Your Mate

Working out with your partner may or may not improve your motivation and performance. It can bring you closer together if you stay aware of the sensitivities involved. It might be better to learn something new together than doing something only one of you is skilled at. Be sure to choose activities the both of you will enjoy. For instance, if one of you hates the cold, don't go skiing.

Turn Your Neighbourhood into a Health Club

You won't pay any dues, and you won't be waiting in any lines by simply going out the door and walking your way into fitness. All you need is a well-designed athletic shoe. Make sure it comes with the proper cushioning. Choose clothing that allows for freedom of movement and remains comfortable in all kinds of weather. If you exercise at night, be sure to wear reflective fabric or attach reflective tape to ensure that you're visible to traffic.

Set Realistic Goals

It could be as simple as firing your housekeeper, and doing your own housework (that's what singer Diana Ross, Eartha Kitt, and others who can easily afford help do to work out). Perhaps it will be walking your dog more often, or just taking the stairs at work instead of using the lift.

You're Already Exercising

Almost everybody walks somewhere. The easiest way to start seeing results is to turn up the voltage on what you normally do. Add a weighted vest or hand weights if possible. You'll feel absolutely pumped!

The Proper Way to Walk

1. Pull your chin in so that your ears are over your shoulders.

2. Relax your shoulders.

3. Concentrate on pulling your tummy in tight.

4. Walk with your arms bent at a 90-degree angle.

5. Tuck your elbows in close to your waist.

6. Try landing strongly on your heels with your toes slightly lifted for a more powerful push off.

7. Let your fingers relax.

8. Hold your wrists straight.

9. Breathe in deeply.

10. Your stride should feel controlled and smooth.

11. Keep your head up.

12. Your eyes should be straight ahead.

13. Be sure not to lean too far forward or back.

14. Let your arms swing naturally.

Walking for Health

Researchers have found that walking for an hour a day decreases the risk of colon cancer by half. Walking speeds digested foods through the body. As a result, toxins in foods spend less time in contact with the colon wall.

Make Your Own Ab Machine
Get a bath towel and lie with it lengthwise
under you. Hold an upper corner of the towel
in each hand. The towel will support your
head and neck while you do sit-ups and
abdominal crunches.

Take It to the Kitchen
Soup cans, drink bottles, and milk cartons make great weights.
Use a sturdy kitchen step-stool to do buttock- and thigh-
strengthening step-ups.

If You Think You're Too Tired
Working out actually boosts your energy for long days, and
helps you cope with stress. It also helps you sleep better. If you
don't feel like exercising, tell yourself you'll just do 5 minutes
instead of 30 minutes. Once you start, you'll probably want to
keep going.

Get a Workout in Your Garden
If you hate sit-ups, the treadmill, and gyms, then get right to
your garden. You can get the same benefits. Here's what to do:

Arms: heavy weeding and composting

Chest: digging and hoeing

Stomach: turning compost and raking

Legs: raking, hoeing, and digging

Back: raking and lawn mowing

Buttocks: weeding, digging, and mowing

Gardening just every other day will make a major difference in
how you look and feel, and don't forget that gardening is known

for giving spiritual nourishment. Spending just 30 minutes in the garden will burn off 150 calories.

Get a Skipping Rope

Your childhood toy may just be the most effective piece of exercise equipment you could own. You've seen those incredibly fit boxers in training. You've seen them jumping away to shape and tone their arms and legs, as well as cutting fat. Skipping will burn fat, define muscles, and is one of the best cures for cellulite. Plus, it's fun, especially if you can remember some of your childhood skipping tunes.

"I like to bring a skipping rope with me when I go for a power walk. I tie it around my waist, and since I walk where there are a lot of traffic lights, I skip while waiting to cross the street."

Sara, age 33, 28 pounds lost

Run if You Can

Even running short distances can yield great health benefits. Running just 15 minutes will burn 150 calories. Running up to 50 miles a week will yield high levels of HDL (good) cholesterol. Runners at this level also have half the rate of hypertension.

Dance Your Fat Away

Get your favourite tunes out and break a sweat! Tap dancing burns 400 calories an hour. The polka will take off 540 calories an hour. Swing dancing burns 300 calories an hour.

"My housework goes by a lot faster — and I exercise — when I put on my old school tunes. It seems like 'yesterday once more' when my stereo wails out those Beatles and Rolling Stones tunes."

Linda, age 47, 34 pounds lost

"I'm a very private person, but I love to dance. When everyone leaves the house, I become that disco diva and get my 30 minutes of exercise."

Ann, age 38, 40 pounds lost

Burn Fat without Trying

Brushing your teeth burns 140 calories a week.

Talking on the phone burns 2 calories a minute.

Playing cards burns 100 calories an hour.

Quality, Not Quantity

More is not always better, especially when you're doing an exercise incorrectly. Be sure to perform each movement slowly and in a controlled manner. Make sure you're in proper body form.

A Little Romance Takes Off

Dancing cheek-to-cheek for one hour burns 200 calories.

Machinery

Although no machine can miraculously give you tighter abs or lift that butt, you may be more motivated if you see it staring you in the face every time you walk into a room. If you're really interested in investing in a machine, you need to ask yourself the following questions:

How much should I spend?

Consider a second-hand piece of equipment if you can't afford a high-quality brand.

Will it fit?

One of the biggest problems is getting a piece of equipment home and discovering it won't go into the closet or even through the door.

"I set up my stair stepper with no problem. But when I went to use it, I found that my head kept hitting the ceiling. What a waste!"

Ben, age 46, 33 pounds lost

Will I really use it?

Even if you hate gyms, and the reason you're buying the equipment is to stay away from them, go for a few sessions. Get a guest pass if you can. See what machines you most enjoy. It might be too embarrassing to try out a piece of equipment in the store. Plus, you really won't get the entire picture if you just spend a minute or two using the demo model.

Stationary Cycles

Look for features like smooth pedalling and a comfortable seat. A stationary cycle is a good idea if cycling is your favourite workout and you want to keep up your routine during the cold winter months. Then when the weather breaks, you're in perfect cycling condition. There are many versions that fold down to a compact size.

Treadmills

Before you plop down your money, be aware that this is the most boring piece of machinery you could buy. Think about it. You're going to run in the same spot every single day. However, a treadmill is a great option if you don't like to run in rain or snow, or if there's an unfriendly dog that has decided to move into the neighbourhood.

Steppers

Look for higher hand grips, which make it a lot harder to "cheat" by leaning on the handrails. It should also allow you to climb at quick pace without sliding backwards. Look for pedals that move independently of each other. This will provide a more challenging workout. A wide stepping area is also desirable because it will be a lot more comfortable. Some of the steppers can be very noisy, so be careful if you enjoy listening to music while you work out.

Rowers

Look for steel or aluminum parts. They will provide longer wear. There is some maintenance involved, and a chain pulling system will mean less work. Toe straps should be very sturdy to be completely comfortable. Look for a rower that provides a smooth ride and a comfortable seat. Some of the models come with a race programme, complete with an imaginary rower. Several models also include a back draft feature. All should feature distance and rowing pace, as well as a timer. Calories-burned estimations sometimes are featured.

Strength Gyms

Look for floating bearings on all moving parts. This makes the machine superior to steel-on-steel construction. These machines should use aircraft-quality nylon-coated cable to connect the weight stacks to each station.

Cross Trainer

This machine is a cross between a bike and a treadmill. Look for resistance settings that can be changed. You might find this machine useful if you're recovering from a sports injury, or you can't take a lot of stress on your joints.

Machine Alternatives

It's not necessary to spend a lot on pricey equipment. You already have tools in your home that can make your workouts more effective.

Chairs

A simple straight-back chair can be used as an exercise tool.
Here are three easy exercises:

> ### Thigh Trimmer
>
> Sit on the edge of a sturdy chair. If possible,
> use ankle weights. Slowly straighten and lift
> one leg, then the other. While the leg is lifted,
> hold to a count of five. Repeat ten to fifteen
> times for each leg.

To Firm Up Hamstrings

Stand straight and hold the back of the chair for balance.

With one leg, slowly lift your heel towards your buttocks. Hold
for a count of five.

Return to starting position, then repeat with other leg.

Repeat ten times for each leg.

You should feel this in the back of your legs.

For Chest and Arms

Sit on the floor with your arms holding the chair's seat.

Extending legs in front of you, raise and lower yourself.

Exhale on the way up, and inhale on the way down.

Repeat ten times.

Books

A thick phone book or encyclopedia can work for several
exercises, including popular "step" work.

To Shape Up Calves

Stand with your toes on a book, holding on to a wall or counter.

Slowly let your heels down as far as you can, feeling the stretch.

Rise again and hold to the count of five.

Repeat ten to fifteen times.

Scarves

Find a sturdy scarf that is at least a square yard in size for this exercise.

Tones Lower Back and Obliques

Stand straight, holding one end of the scarf in each hand.

Raise arms and pull scarf hard.

Twist the body as far to the right, and as far to the left as you can.

Do this ten to fifteen times.

Vegetable Cans

Vegetable and soup cans make perfect small weights for these toning exercises.

Pecs Enhancer

Create great cleavage by toning your pectoral muscles.

Hold a vegetable can in each hand. Lift your arms straight out to the side, with elbows slightly bent.

Bring your arms to the front of your body until the cans touch.

Repeat fifteen times.

No More Flabby Arms

Taking a vegetable can in one hand, lean over a chair and place your other hand on the seat.

Fully extend the arm holding the vegetable can and reach backwards and up.

Do this twenty times with each arm.

You'll know you should be doing this exercise if your arm still waves "good-bye" after you stop.

The Wall

Use the wall as a resistance tool.

"Kiss the Wall"

Stand about three feet from a wall, back straight, legs bent slightly at the knee.

Extend your arms straight in front of you, and rest your palms against the wall.

Bending your arms, lower your body towards the wall and "kiss" it.

Push yourself back and repeat twenty times.

Bottle Beauties

1. Stand with your knees slightly bent, and grip a two-litre bottle. Keeping elbows close to the side, move lower arm up and down. Repeat ten times with each arm.
2. For great shoulders lift bottles in front of you. Keep elbows and knees slightly bent. Move bottle to your eye level. Repeat twenty times.
3. Hold bottles at sides and bend knees and elbows. Slowly raise arms out to the sides up to the ears. Repeat twenty times.

Broomstick

A great tool for balance and lifting.

Stationary Lunge

Holding on to the top of the broomstick, step back with left foot.

Bend knees and drop hips until left shin is parallel to the floor.

Both knees should be at right angles.

Rise from lunge position, lifting knee to a 90-degree angle.

Alternate legs and repeat fifteen times.

Hey! Great Shoulders!

Developing your upper back will make you look like you've lost five pounds!

No More Excuses

Time

Think of the time you waste each day. It may be on the phone, flicking through TV channels, or browsing the shops. You can always find time when it's important to you. Even if you have to set your alarm 30 minutes earlier, make the time.

Injury

Of course, certain physical conditions prevent exercising. Most problems, however, can be worked around. A physical therapist can set up a programme that's safe and effective for you.

Video Hype

With so many exercise videos on the market today, how do you tell what's going to work without wasting a lot of money? Here's a few things to look for:

1. Inspect the claims and don't fall for the "pie in the sky" promises.

2. Look for credentials. Check out certification, and don't fall for vague titles like "America's best fitness trainer".

3. Find the copyright date. New data on training pops up every

day. Don't buy anything that's more than two years old.

4. See what else you might need. You might bring home a tape and find out that it's to be used with an ab roller and you don't own or want one.

5. Don't fall for lingo. If the box is not easy to understand, you won't be able to follow along with the video.

Chapter Nine

Intimacy and Weight

It's All about Self-Perception
Both men and women relate weight with not feeling sexual or seductive. Women especially blame themselves for not fitting into society's so-called physical ideal of seductiveness. Yet most people do not and cannot fit into the ideal of the fashion magazines and screen (TV and movies) images. There is no data available to indicate that size has any effect on seductiveness.

So You're Not a Supermodel
Not many people are, but everyone's trying to look like one. Sex is not about how you look, it's about how you feel.

A Happy Love Life Can Help
Don't use the excuse that you don't have a perfect body to avoid sex. Sex can help you look and feel better. Just think of it as one of the more pleasant ways to lose weight.

Sex Is Good Exercise
Believe it or not, an amorous lovemaking session will burn off 500 calories in an hour. Hey, that's about as much as 40 minutes on a treadmill!

Sex Lowers Cholesterol
Scientists have found that your body's cholesterol level drops

after a lovemaking session.

Sex Regulates Menstruation
If you are a victim of irregular menstrual cycles, check your sex life. Researchers have found that women who have sex every week are more likely to have regular menstrual cycles of 28 or 29 days.

Better Skin Tone
People who have sex regularly find that their skin tone is better, due to the level of hormones being raised. It may be the reason people who are in love look so radiant. These increased levels of hormones are also known to cause hair to grow faster and give it extra shine.

No More Headache Excuses
Throw away the aspirin. Hormones released during sex, such as progesterone, act as a mild anaesthetic, easing pain and headaches.

Sex Can Make You Smarter
During sex the oxygen level in the blood is raised. This has an energising effect on the muscles, and revs up mental ability.

Surprising Scents That Put You in the Mood
Pumpkin pie
Licorice
Doughnuts (mostly men)

Hygiene Is Most Important
Both men and women mentioned body odour as being their number one sexual turn off. No matter what your size, it has the most lasting negative impression. It is especially important to shower daily if you are very far from your final weight goal.

Fake It

No, I'm not getting that personal, and I don't mean to suggest you fake anything involved with the sex act itself. What I mean is that you should act like you are a godsend to the opposite sex and soon you'll begin to really feel that way. If you find yourself unattractive, so will everyone else.

"Even though I was a size fourteen, I was ashamed that I was not a size four. I rarely dated, and when I did, my dates never failed to comment on my weight. My best friend, who was two sizes bigger than I was at the time, not only had more dates than me, but also had a couple of marriage proposals. Unlike me, she was totally happy being a size eighteen. She had been a woman of size all her life, and walked into a room like she owned it. Even when I finally got down to a size eight, I still couldn't attract the type of guy I wanted. It was only through therapy that I was able to figure out that it had little to do with weight."

Rachel, age 40, 53 pounds lost

Don't Squeeze

Wearing clothing that is too tight is constricting and bothersome. You will feel more sexually confident with flowing clothes that feel good on your body. It will change the way you feel, and even the way you walk. Practise walking in front of the mirror the way models do. Put one foot in front of the other, toes and balls of your feet before your heels, head held high. Tuck your tummy in and pull your shoulders back. This will make you look pounds thinner, taller, and you'll look and feel sexier. Walking a little faster will also get people to notice you.

Work Out Together

Grunting and sweating together is sexy! If you aren't physically up to a big workout, just taking a walk together will help you connect.

117

> ## Your Body Is Not a Weapon
>
> Don't use it as one against your partner. Some dieters I talked to told me that they actually gained weight in order to create a buffer. They put on the pounds because they knew that their partner would be upset about it. The result is that the dieter became even more unhappy.

"My girlfriend and I are pretty competitive. When we started working out together it became our favourite foreplay."

Ken, age 27, 25 pounds lost

"I took my husband for a surprise hike on a very secluded path. We took some breaks."

Alexis, age 25, 30 pounds lost

Discover Self-Love

Look in the mirror, smile, and just say "hi!" Self-acceptance is harder when there's no feedback coming from outside sources. The more desperate we become for compliments and reaffirmation, the harder it will be to lose the weight. Concentrate on something you see in the mirror that you like, rather than your short-comings. If you have great hair, an engaging smile, or shapely legs, you have a tool that is significant to your self-esteem as well as to your sensuality.

"When I went from 125 to 185 pounds, I lost total confidence in myself. I felt completely useless and nonsexual. I pushed my husband away, in every way, even though he never sent me any negative vibes. I became reclusive, combative, and we eventually divorced."

Susan, age 32, 50 pounds lost

Celery, The Great Seducer

Men who have been practising their best lines for seduction should shut up and start chewing. Scientists have found that the potent male hormone androsterone is found in celery. Androsterone is released through perspiration after eating. Although the smell of celery itself is undetectable, the hormone has the power to attract women. Side benefits include a high-fibre, low-calorie snack that freshens breath.

Coffee, The No-Calorie Turn On

Studies indicate that our morning cup of coffee may not only be getting us going, but turning us on. Men and women who have at least one cup of coffee a day are nearly twice as likely to describe themselves as sexually active. Men who drink coffee reportedly have less problems with erections.

Create Flattering Lighting

Certain lighting can bring flattering reflection to the skin tone. Photographers know this, and you can use it if you're less than confident about your body. Replace your lighting with pink- or blue-tinted light bulbs in your bedroom. A 20-watt incandescent bulb will do wonders! If you can't find any of these bulbs in your hardware or drugstore, just light a few candles.

Foods for Passion

There are foods that not only will help you lose those extra pounds, but will get you in the mood.

Apples

Remember what happened to Adam and Eve?

Bananas

Known as the fruit of love, the banana is revered in Asia and Africa. They are rich in potassium and B6, associated with female sex hormones.

Cinnamon
Known throughout the ages as an important romantic enhancement.

Dill
Use it as a tea, add it to breads or salads, or just eat a pickle.

Eggs
Folklore claims that eggs can cure sexual diseases. Today we know that they're rich in an essential amino acid that influences sexual arousal.

Figs
Rich in niacin and magnesium.

Ginseng
Very popular today, it was known in China to keep men virile. Take it as a capsule, drink it as a tea, or visit a Chinese super-market for other foods.

Green Tea
Said to strengthen body fluids.

Honey Pollen
Stimulates the reproductive system. Add it to yoghurt or cottage cheese.

Lavender
It can be added to sauces and desserts.

Lemons
Supposedly adds staying power.

Mussels
It could be just a visual, but it's been a constant. Plus it's rich in iron.

Mushrooms
They are great by themselves, added to antipasto, broiled, or marinated.

Nutmeg
A little goes a long way as a sugar substitute.

Oysters
Rich in zinc, they are undoubtedly the favourite aphrodisiac — and with good reason.

Parsley
It also gives you fresh breath for kissing! Almost NO calories here.

Peaches
The fruit of passion for their suggestive shape and soft touch. A great source of vitamin A, which manufactures sex hormones.

Raspberries
Another vitamin A source.

Scallops
Makes for sensual eating, and is very low in calories.

Sunflower Seeds
A good source of phosphorus directly impacting sexual desire.

Wine
Just a little as a spritzer. Too much is too many calories and will put you to sleep.

Chapter Ten

Holidays, Vacations and other Trip-Ups

You Can Handle Those Special Occasions

There's no need to turn down an invitation, cancel a trip, or avoid an important family celebration because of fear of gaining weight. Just because you've made the decision to lose weight doesn't mean you have to deprive yourself of life's pleasures. You can't push life away while you diet. Even if you're at your healthy weight, you have to learn to handle yourself in the everyday circumstances of life. However, even the most disciplined dieter can become completely overwhelmed by the events and situations that take us from our everyday routine. Temptations, family pressure, and just plain inconvenience can undermine willpower and discipline. Here's how winners in the weight-loss game overcame these difficult situations.

Christmas

There's no reason to dread Christmas. It should be a favourite time of the year. There's enough stress with shopping, house cleaning, and scheduling time and people. Healthy living means moderation, not deprivation. Keep the traditions and foods of the season you've come to love by making some minor modifications. Be sure to remember the true spirit of the day. Family, friendship, and love are what this holiday means. It's not about pies, cakes, and biscuits. Concentrate on the true spirit.

Food is important, of course, but it's not what you truly want to remember about this holiday.

Turkey

White meat is lower in fat than dark meat. Five ounces of sliced, skinless white meat contains 219 calories. Five ounces of sliced, skinless dark meat has 262 calories. Also, substituting turkey drippings with a gravy base made from chicken broth will cut calories in half.

"I substitute maple syrup for butter to glaze the turkey. Then I baste it with some of the turkey drippings. It's delicious!"

Sally, age 44, 50 pounds lost

Mashed Potatoes

"We love mashed potatoes, but the calories are killer! I made a few changes to lower them by blending skimmed milk instead of whole and adding garlic to season. My family loved it, and I saved ten grams of fat from the original recipe."

Mary, age 48, 33 pounds lost

Stuffing

"Rather than the traditional stuffing baked inside the turkey itself, I make a cornbread stuffing that I moisten with broth. It doesn't taste greasy, and yet it's not too dry."

Pat, age 34, 40 pounds lost

Make an Allowance

Save your fat calories if you've been dreaming about your sister's quiche. Eat lightly at other meals, concentrating on fruits and vegetables.

"If I know that I'm going to a big holiday party, I prepare myself by eating salads for dinner all week, and passing on too many snacks. Not only do I have the calorie allotment for that 'special' meal, but I look better in my holiday outfit."

Ann, age 38, 40 pounds lost

Be a Good Guest

Offer to bring a dish, and make it a delicious recipe that's also low in calories. You'll be a hero for helping out a busy host, and you'll have something you know that you can eat without trepidation.

"When I go to a party, I try to prepare myself before I go. I look over the table, and if I don't see anything I can eat, I just grab a beverage and get into the conversation. If I think I'm being watched, I put a couple of things on my plate and kind of move it around."

Dina, age 39, 25 pounds lost

When It's Your Party

Although you have the control here, you want to serve food that will really be enjoyed by your guests. If you only put out a bunch of celery sticks and carrots, it's going to make for some quick exits. Create a combination of choices so everyone there will find something to enjoy. That said, you can substitute skimmed milk for whole, egg beaters for whole eggs, etc., and your guests won't even notice.

Don't Eat the Decorations

It's festive to use sweets, candied fruits, nuts, cheese balls, and other condiments to decorate the house. They seem to lurk at every corner, and are easy to scoop up as you pass by. Instead, use scented sachets, pine cones, and primitive crafts that are inedible.

"Our family traditionally decorated the tree with candy canes that we eventually ate. Now we string popcorn and cranberry chains."

Ginger, age 51, 30 pounds lost

Gift Giving

A lot of food gifts are passed around this time of year because something homemade is definitely a more meaningful display of affection. But your delicious homemade biscuits may not be appreciated by a calorie-conscious recipient. Make an arrangement of dried flowers, a simple pine cone wreath, or framed picture. Not only will it be just as meaningful, but it's a gift that will be a long-lasting remembrance.

Portion Control

It's not the food itself that's bad for you, but the excessive portions that are consumed. Having a little of everything is a good way to ensure that nobody's feelings are hurt, and you won't deprive yourself of different tastes.

"Before I head to a holiday party, I have a bowl of high-fibre cereal with a large glass of water. It doesn't weigh me down, and yet gives me a sense of control so that I don't eat everything I see."

Mac, age 35, 58 pounds lost

Don't Pick

Put your entire meal on one plate so that you know just how much you are eating. Seconds are not an option. Wash it all down with water or a diet beverage. Even better, carry a toothbrush and brush your teeth to indicate to your mind and mouth that you are done.

Buffets

Going to a party that features a buffet can actually be a blessing in disguise. You can survive without the scrutiny that would occur if you were seated. Plus, since you're moving around, the food isn't "in your face" where temptation will be at its full force.

> ### Use Fibre
> Bake biscuits with added fibre, like oat bran.
> This will greatly cut the calorie content, and will
> make the biscuit more filling.

Scan the Table

Look around the buffet table for items that still somewhat resemble the whole foods from which they were derived. Look for dishes based on vegetables, fruits, and grains. Avoid thick sauces and gravy-laden dishes. Fill your plate with fresh vegetables and salads.

Limit Yourself to One Trip

The danger of the buffet is that you may never stop eating. Resolve that you will make one trip, and that you will eat slowly while everyone else is making their third and fourth trip back.

Choose a Small Plate

Take the smallest plate available, and then pile it on. You'll fool yourself into thinking that you're having a big meal. Leave the smallest part of the plate for the food you should have the least of.

Eat Your Favourite Foods First

The food that catches your eye first is the one that you should eat first. That's the secret of the perpetually thin person.

> ### Pass on the Ordinary
>
> Don't bother to eat what you regularly eat all year. This is the time to enjoy those special foods. Remember this: the first one you eat makes it special. After that, the pleasure is reduced by about 50 percent, and it goes down even further

Go Fish

Shrimp, scallops, crab, and salmon are common buffet fare that are all very low in fat. They'll keep you away from the meatballs and cocktail franks.

Buffet Bites

1. Stick with lean meats or grilled foods.
2. If you love cheese, eat chunks of it and stay away from the spreads.
3. Bean dips contain less calories than sour cream varieties.
4. Salsa is fat-free and a dieter's dream. It usually has only ten calories for two big tablespoons.
5. Choose wholegrain crackers over crisps.

Buffet Calorie Count

Buffalo chicken wing = 254 calories
Celery stalk = 6 calories
Cocktail meatball = 20 calories
Whole carrot = 3 calories
Scoop of nuts = 55 calories
Stuffed mushroom = 80 calories

Potato crisp with dip = 21 calories
Teaspoon of caviar = 15 calories
One shrimp or scallop = 10 calories
Five Ritz crackers with 1 ounce pâté = 200 calories
Three bite-size bacon quiches = 300 calories
Brie in pastry = 230 calories
Eight medium strawberries = 50 calories

Concentrate on People

The fun of a buffet is that it's for mingling, not munching. Move around with a glass of seltzer with lime in your hand and get caught up with the crowd. If you're the hostess, try to have a mingling area that does not involve food. Set up a table with a jigsaw puzzle that all the party goers will attempt to put together.

Low-Calorie Party Mix

Oat square cereal
Miniature cinnamon rice cakes
Raisins
Low-fat pretzels

Mix together in a festive bowl.

"A great way to prevent a host from bugging me all night to overeat is to take a little bite, and then rave about how delicious the dish is. The reaction is appreciated by the host, and then they move on to somebody else."

Nick, age 67, 38 pounds lost

Alcohol

Those liquid calories can quickly add up. Alcohol is greatly to blame for the extra calories consumed at special events.

Alcohol with Water

Have one glass of water with every glass of alcohol you drink. By alternating between alcohol and water you'll cut your calories in half. Alcohol stimulates appetite, so be aware that as you drink, your willpower will go down.

Watch Those Calories

Research indicates that those alcoholic beverages you're enjoying tonight will turn up as fat tomorrow. These calories are metabolised like fat. There is a way to counteract this effect. By eating magnesium-rich foods like lean cuts of meat, dark green leafy vegetables, and wholegrain products, you will control your body's response to the sugar effect of alcohol. Some people actually take magnesium supplements to normalise their body's response to these sugars when they drink.

Smart Choices

White wine = 80 calories
Light beer = 100 calories
Champagne = 75 calories
Vodka with cranberry juice = 125 calories

Bad Choices

Eggnog = 275 calories
Brandy Alexander = 305 calories
White Russian = 235 calories
Pina colada = 265 calories

Space It Out

If you space out your drinking to one alcoholic beverage every hour, it greatly cuts down your amount of overindulging not only in alcohol, but it keeps your willpower in check so that you don't overeat.

If You Overdid It

A bartender I know swears this is what you can do that "morning after" you drank too much. Take a shot of vodka, a squirt of lemon, and a drop of Tabasco. Dissolve a beef bouillon in 1/2 cup of warm water. Add it all together, and drink away that hangover.

Valentine's Day

We all know that roses contain a lot less calories than a box of chocolates. But it's OK to indulge from time to time. Here's the calorie count on some of the traditional favourites.

Chocolate candy heart = 69 calories
2 cherry cordials = 180 calories
Candy conversation hearts (1 ounce) = 110 calories

Don't forget the champagne. Two glasses of the sparkly stuff will set you back by only 150 calories. Champagne contains half the calories of sweet wine and one-third the calories of hard liquor. It also aids digestion with its natural carbon gas, magnesium, and potassium.

Easter

Raiding the Easter basket can be dangerous, so dig into those fat-free jelly beans. They are the best sweet in the loot. Each bean contains only about 5 or 6 calories.

Dining Out

Eating in a restaurant can become creative combat in any diet programme. However, with these little steps, it can be a pleasant break from a boring routine without costing a lot of calories.

Don't Arrive Famished

Have a few glasses of water with lemon and a few carrot sticks before heading out.

The World's Best-Kept Diet Secrets

Save the Alcohol for the Meal

If you enjoy any kind of alcohol when you are dining out, have it during your meal, not before. Alcohol is a high-calorie beverage and can stimulate your appetite. It can also impair your judgement about food choices. After all, drinks, especially wines, can enhance the enjoyment of the meal.

Leave Out the Bread Basket

Ask that the breads arrive with the meal, otherwise you'll make a meal out of its contents. If you're truly hungry, order an appetiser that takes work to eat. A good choice would be steamed clams or escargot.

Lead the Conversation

Talk a lot during the meal. You can't make polite conversation with your mouth full of food, so let your personality become the table's entertainment.

Cuisine Choices

	Order	Avoid
American	Poultry and seafood	Fatty meats
	Grilled meats	Fried fish
	Vegetables and salads	Dressings
Chinese	Broth-based soups	Fried noodles, egg rolls
	Steamed fish, vegetables	Egg foo yung
	Chop suey and stir fry	Battered dishes
	White rice	Duck
French	Steamed mussels	Vichyssoise
	Poached seafood	Quiche
	Seafood/poultry in parchment	Heavy creams (like Remoulade)
	Parfait	Mousse

Greek	Bean and lentil soups	Spanakopita
	Shish kebab	Feta cheese
	Baked fish (Plaki)	Moussaka
	Orzo	Baklava
Italian	Vegetable soup	Antipasto
	Seafood stew (Cioppino)	Fried calamari
	Pasta with vegetables	Pasta with heavy sauce
	Baked or broiled polenta	Marinated vegetables
Mexican	Steamed tortillas	Nachos
	Black and pinto beans	Refried beans
	Salsa	Guacamole
	Gazpacho	Enchilada

Travel

Battling the bulge while travelling is not as difficult as you may believe. It starts when you make your reservations and will make a positive difference in your energy and stress levels. It just takes a little creativity and some advance planning sprinkled in with a little discipline.

> Diners are most likely to eat foolishly during the first ten minutes of a social gathering.

Do Some Leg Work

Phone your hotel and ask about gym facilities on site or nearby. Inquire about nearby parks, running tracks, hiking trails, tennis courts, and other exercising options. Ask if there are shuttle services to some of these areas. Even shuttles to shopping areas are good for a spirited mall walk.

Make Reservations

Call your airline and ask about special meals. Every airline will offer an alternative, and your best bet is vegetarian or low fat. Some even offer cold seafood, all fruit, and Hindu (a baked potato and steamed vegetables).

Packing

Tuck a skipping rope into your suitcase. You can use it on carpeting or outdoors. Travel with your favourite exercise tape. Hotels that offer convention services will have VCRs that are available for guest use. Pack a pair of walking/running shoes, and fold in an exercise elastic band for resistance work.

Driving

Practise isometrics at traffic lights. Squeeze your buttocks and hold for a count of ten. Raise your lower lip, trying to touch your nose to improve jaw line definition.

At the Airport

Airport delays are frustrating both to the mind and body. Overeating at a food court can result from sheer boredom. Instead, take advantage of the time by walking as fast and as far as you can. If you have lots of "stuff" that would weigh you down, there are convenient lockers located throughout. Some airports have even started installing day gyms.

In the Air

Request an exit row or bulkhead seat. You'll have more comfort and room to move. Take advantage of headphones, and look for the channels with upbeat music. Do some easy leg stretches and move your arms around. Circulation can suffer on long trips.

While in Your Seat

1. Flex your ankles and work your calf muscles.

2. Do seated calf raises with your paperwork (or a child) on your lap.

In the Aisle

1. Grab each ankle and pull your heel up to your buttocks. Hold for a count of ten and alternate.

2. Try to touch your toes while waiting for the lavatory to stretch your hamstrings.

3. Reach up towards the ceiling, alternating hands. Do this ten times.

At Your Hotel

1. Refuse the key to your mini-bar to avoid temptation.

2. Check with your concierge about safe walking or jogging areas.

3. Stage some workouts in the hotel's pool. The natural buoyancy causes the muscles to work harder, and it feels just great.

4. See if your hotel has access to bike rentals.

5. You don't need to pack your weights. Every hotel has books and lamps.

The Mummy Track

It's not necessary to put your diet and fitness routines on hold because there are little ones around. Your kids can help you become more active and fit.

Sports

Find a sport that the whole family can enjoy. Biking (very safe and comfortable models are available) and hiking are sports for kids of every age. Babies love the new running strollers on the market which allow you to power walk/run.

A Natural Weight

Mums get a great upper arm workout by lifting little ones over their shoulders and above their heads.

Videos

Check out the video tapes specially created for parent and child bonding.

> ### Health Clubs
>
> There's nothing better than an hour reprieve, and you'll be more at ease if you check out gyms and health clubs that offer on-site baby-sitting services. Separation anxiety? Choose a club where the child centre is in your view.

Chapter Eleven

Other Weight-Loss Options

Beyond Dieting

There are options in losing weight that go beyond cutting down on calories. Sometimes dieting and exercise alone cannot engender total satisfaction in one's body. There are techniques that are considered short cuts and final solutions. Some are controversial, while others are risky.

Liposuction

The number one requested cosmetic surgery procedure today is liposuction, the suctioning of excess fat from certain areas of the body. Certain body types carry pockets of fat that just can't be exercised off. It is a procedure that has only been around since the early eighties. When it was originally introduced, the fluid that was extracted was about half fat and half blood. Now, there are new, safer methods that remove almost 100 per cent fat alone. Still, it is the informed patients who report the best results. Cosmetic surgery is still major surgery.

Risks

There are very rare reports of complications that can come from any surgery. They include infection, blood clots (sometimes fatal), reactions to anaesthesia, or perforation to the skin or organs caused by improper probing or excess force. This is the result of excessive instrument force by inexperienced surgeons.

Candidates
An ethical surgeon will not perform liposuction as a weight-loss alternative. The ideal candidate for liposuction should be near a healthy weight for their body type and age.

Who Performs Liposuction?
Liposuction techniques are now being performed by dermatologic surgeons, cosmetic surgeons, and plastic surgeons. Both dermatologic surgeons and plastic surgeons are currently being taught liposuction during their residency training programmes.

Body Areas
The most frequently treated areas are the waistline, abdomen, inner and outer thighs (saddlebags), buttocks, knees, ankles, and neck area. Men are now getting liposuction in the breast area.

Ultrasonic Liposuction
This technique uses sound waves to liquefy the fat. The procedure is less invasive than traditional liposuction, making recovery time a lot quicker. Many surgeons are even performing this procedure in their offices or in an ambulatory surgery centre. With this procedure, blood loss is greatly reduced.

Gastric Surgery
Surgery to treat chronic or severe obesity grew out of the results of operations for cancer and severe ulcers. It removes large portions of the stomach or small intestine. The result was that these procedures resulted in large weight losses following the surgery. Surgeons, recognising the results, began using it to treat patients with a lot of weight to lose as long as 40 years ago. Patients are not considered for this operation unless they are at least 100 pounds overweight or have a body mass index (BMI) of 40 or above. A weight problem must be severe, or even life-threatening, to be considered.

How It Works
The surgery limits how much the stomach can hold. The patient is able to make better food choices and experience satiety that may not have been able to be assuaged previously. Food intake is restricted because for most people the ability to eat a large amount of food is gone. Usually, only one-half to a whole cup of food can be eaten at one time without severe discomfort.

Risks
A small percentage of patients required follow-up surgery to correct complications. Abdominal hernias were the most common complication, but also included were breakdown of the staple line and stretched stomach outlets. Some patients had problems with gallstones. This was the result of losing weight rapidly, which can occur with any quick weight loss.

Other problems included nutritional deficiencies such as anaemia, osteoporosis, and metabolic bone disease. These problems are preventable if vitamin and mineral supplements are taken after surgery. A small percentage of the patients had a problem with vomiting. This was caused by overstretching of the stomach by food particles that had not been chewed thoroughly. Less than 1 per cent of complications resulted in death.

Success Rate
Research reports that about 30 per cent of patients are able to get to a normal weight after this surgery. About 80 per cent of patients achieved some degree of weight loss. The problem with this surgery is that some patients are unable to adjust their eating habits. Some surgeons require behaviour modification follow-up on their patients. The real success reported by this type of operation was a commitment to a lifelong change in eating and long-term medical monitoring. This is a complicated procedure, only to be used as a profound last measure, and should be carefully researched.

Body Lifts

These are "face lifts" for the thighs, buttocks, hips, and stomach. The procedure smooths and tightens sagging skin that has lost its elasticity, many times due to excess weight loss.

How It Works

A section of the skin is removed (sometimes after liposuction), and a section of the fibres and muscles beneath it are tightened. The remaining skin is pulled taut and stitched together. Sometimes it is the only way to get rid of cellulite for good.

Cons

Extensive scars are the biggest disadvantage to this type of operation. It's also very expensive, and about five times more costly than liposuction. Since it's major surgery, the risks involving anaesthesia, etc. also exist. In some cases, a blood transfusion may be necessary. Recovery time is also somewhat lengthy.

Other Weight-Related Surgeries

Tummy Tuck

This surgery removes excess fat or skin that may have been stretched by pregnancy or obesity. It is performed under general anaesthesia and involves several days of hospitalisation. There is also an extensive recovery period of several weeks. After a lot of weight is lost, successful dieters may be thrilled with their new bodies, but not their sagging tummy area. My interview subjects reported wanting this procedure first and foremost after their weight loss.

> ### Breast Reduction
> Women who are at a normal weight sometimes still felt fat with large breasts. Although losing the weight was a liberating experience, they still reported physical limitations and discomfort caused by oversized breasts. This surgery held the highest satisfaction rate of any of the procedures.

Breast Implants

Due to weight loss, ageing, and breast feeding, breast augmentation is being done with saline and occasionally soy bean implants. Silicone breast implants are now illegal in the United States.

Breast Lift

Another surgery that many times follows weight loss. A breast lift raises and shapes droopy breasts. There is some visible scarring from this surgery.

Male Breast Reduction

This is a little talked about operation. Many times excessive breast tissue in men can be reduced with liposuction. Sometimes, although the breasts in men are not bigger, it can appear that way as a result of a large weight loss. In this case, the surgeon will remove the excess skin.

Cellulite Treatments

I have been witness to the thinnest person dieting away in an attempt to get rid of cellulite. Cellulite is hereditary, and it is not necessarily the result of heavy legs and thighs. I've seen 90-pound anorexic models with cellulite. There are many treatments available today, most of which can be used at home.

Acids

There are a myriad of acid-based creams on the market today. The acids speed up natural exfoliation, making dimply skin look smoother. Look for percentages in the 12 to 15 per cent range. Or to get a natural acid without the chemicals, use milk. Powdered milk is lactic acid. Make a thick paste by adding a little water to the powder and massage it into the affected area. Use a rough washcloth or a loofah, as it's half the art of the massage that works on cellulite.

Caffeine

The way caffeine gets us up and going in the morning is the same way it gets those pesky fat cells going. It's the number one ingredient in some of the priciest cellulite creams available today. Save lots of money by doing this spa treatment yourself. Take your warm, used coffee grounds out of your coffee maker. Sitting on the edge of your bathtub with some newspaper underneath to prevent a mess, rub the grounds into your cellulite. Massage it in thoroughly for at least 5 minutes. Wrap your thighs and the coffee residue with plastic wrap. Let it sit and detoxify the skin for at least 10 minutes. Then just rinse it off. You can also use seaweed (found dried in health food stores) and wet it down as an effective wrap. The seaweed will detoxify the skin and draw out any impurities.

Endermologie

A mechanical massager, available only at endermologie centres, is being used to smooth out skin. The concept is that this machine will draw out the cellulite, knead it, and break up the connective fibres. This procedure is costly, and has to be kept up. Usually it's necessary to have this treatment performed on a weekly basis.

Chapter Twelve

Shortcuts

Fit and Fabulous, Fast!

There are the tricks of the trade used by the best bodies around that work quickly and effectively. They are the techniques that come out when time is of the essence. These are the secrets whispered by trainers, agents, and the stars themselves that are the very cutting edge of the industry. By using these little secrets, you'll be amazed at the results.

The Ultimate Jump-Start Diet

The Garlic and Papaya Diet

This is a totally natural diuretic when you need to get into an outfit quickly and safely. Many models use it to prepare for a photo shoot .This is the "secret" formula behind very expensive capsules being sold in Hollywood.

Take two garlic tablets and two papaya tablets before breakfast, lunch, and dinner. These tablets are available in your local drugstore or health food store. Ask your pharmacist for the strongest strength available over the counter. Eat lightly for two days, staying away from salt, bread, and carbonated beverages. Stay near a bathroom because this will draw fluids (safely) from your body.

Iced Water

Ask anybody with a body "to die for," and most likely they will tell you that they drink lots of water. The water is true, but it's only half the story. It's the ice that you add to your water that really makes the difference. Drinking iced water forces your system to rev up your metabolism, keeping the body's temperature from dropping. For example, if you drink eight 12-ounce glasses of iced water a day, your body will burn an additional 200 calories.

Drink water consistently throughout the day. By the time you are really feeling thirsty, you are on your way to becoming dehydrated.

Often what we think of as hunger is thirst. If you find it difficult to down water in large quantities, flavour it up with a bit of lemon or lime. Water can provide a feeling of fullness, and it helps the kidneys and liver do their job.

Don't be fooled into thinking that drinking lots of water will bloat you. Water retention is more likely to be caused by not drinking enough.

Spicy Foods

Scientists have discovered that chilli, peppers, salsa, mustard, and ginger can actually raise your metabolic rate. The result is you can burn calories much faster, up to 45 per cent faster than that of a bland diet. How? These foods create a thermogenic burn, meaning it helps the body to produce "heat", thus burning off calories. Forget all those "thermogenesis" products out there. Just start adding some "spice" into your diet.

> ### Seeds
>
> To maximise your intake of nutrients, add a lot of seed-containing fruits and vegetables such as apples, pears, and bananas, as well as the seeds themselves (like sesame or sunflower seeds). Seeds are a great source of fibre, allowing foods to go through your body

Say It with Soy

Adding soy to your diet will add more than just a fabulous figure. Soy is packed with powerful antioxidants which interfere with free radical damage. This is the basis for how fast we age. Soy is another reason to turn to a more vegetarian-based diet. Unlike animal proteins, soybeans don't spew scads of damaging free radicals through your body to age your cells. Soy also prevents heart disease and diabetes. Japanese, who eat the most soybean in the world (thirty times more than Americans), live longer than anyone. Soy is also reported to cut breast cancer rates and lower blood cholesterol.

Look Buff!

Before you shower or bathe, dry brush your body with a coarse loofah. It will slough off dead cells, stimulate circulation, and aid lymphatic drainage. It will unbloat your body!

Tack a Mirror on It

You can purchase a mirror that attaches to the front of the refrigerator. You'll find that if you have to face yourself each time you peek in, it just may wake you up to reality.

Tape up an Inspirational Note

Make that note a trigger for your success. Try something like, "I can do it" or "Just a month until swimsuit season."

Keep the Fat in the Fridge

Take one pound of butter or shortening and keep it in a plastic bag. Make it the first thing you see when you open that refrigerator.

Portion All Your Foods

Pack all your food in bags. You'll see your daily allotment at a glance. Knowing that you're limited to those bags provides a focus.

Good Foods for Great Looks!

Blueberries

Promote healthy collagen for fewer wrinkles and help create less constriction of veins and faster healing.

Carrots

Contain high levels of beta carotene for protection against sun damage.

Salmon

Rich in essential fatty acids to keep skin moisturised.

Eggs

High in the amino acid "cystein", necessary for the growth and maintenance of the body's tissues.

Yams

Rich in vitamin A to protect the skin from environmental damage.

Mushrooms

Rich in selenium, an antioxidant that may help lower skin cancer risks.

Sugarless Sweets

Sweets and gums sweetened with artificial sweeteners can't be broken down by the body efficiently and can cause severe bloating.

Yoghurt

Contains vitamin B complex, which is essential for smooth, blemish-free skin.

Consider This!

Red Wine

Drinking a glass of red wine can speed up metabolism rates.

Lollipops

Sucking on a lollipop can calm nerves and stop sugar cravings.

Stomachs Can Shrink

After a period of restricting calories, the stomach's capacity will actually decrease.

Tensing

No need to stay at home with an expensive ab machine when you can tense your stomach muscles in and out wherever you are!

The Fat Test

If you want to know if a food is high in fat, but the box isn't around so you can read the labelling, rub the food with a paper napkin. If it leaves a grease mark, it's probably got more fat than you want.

Grow Up!

Start experimenting with exotic foods which are low in calories. For instance, portabello mushrooms are exotic and look like a large steak. Leave those big fat-filled cheeseburgers to the little kids.

Cut Back on Calories without Counting

Eat Your Treats

If you don't treat yourself now and then, you'll just crave it more. It will lead to an unfortunate binge.

Leave Out the Fat

Chances are many of your favourite foods can remain in your diet if you cut back on cheese, butter, cream, etc.

Spread It

Salad dressings, spreads, etc. can be thinned out with vinegars, yoghurt, and other low-fat extenders.

Check Portions

Weigh and measure your foods when it's convenient.

Stop Late-Night Eating
Your body can't digest those late-night snacks when it's at rest.

Don't Drink Calories
Learn to like low-calorie drinks for painless calorie cutting.

What's in Your Coffee?
Since there are so many speciality coffees around, be certain that you're really ordering a potentially delicious, refreshing low-calorie drink.

American drip	4 calories
American decaf	4 calories
Espresso	5 calories
Latte	60 calories
Cappuccino	40 calories
Cafe mocha	150 calories

Don't Skip Meals
You'll end up eating twice as much and your metabolism will be messed up with low blood-sugar levels.

Shop with the Right Attitude
Never go shopping for food when you're ravenous! You'll end up with all the wrong stuff in your trolley.

Proteins for Weight Loss
All proteins are not the same. To lose weight more quickly, eat egg whites, steamed or grilled fish, chicken, and turkey.

Eating as Meditation

Increase your satisfaction by slowing down and stepping inside of yourself. Remove any distractions, focus on your food, and take only what you need. Chew with deep awareness, noting how you feel when you have finished.

Chew Hard

Any fruit or vegetable that is hard to chew delivers better fibre and prevents blood-sugar dips.

Trick Your Body

We all want to sin a little, so stay away from the "all or nothing" syndrome. Replace sugary or fatty snacks with complex carbohydrates and low percentages of fat. No fat foods adds up to no satisfaction.

Sleep More

Studies show that when people don't get enough sleep, they eat more food, and they eat it more often.

Eat It Cold

Foods that are cooled down lose some of their calories and are harder to digest.

Stay Away from Alligators

If a fruit or vegetable has hard skin, it's likely to be higher in calories and fat than smooth-skinned varieties. The reason is its water content. That's why a tomato has a lot less calories than an avocado.

Grate Your Food

Use a grater, and watch your food grow. Carrots, apples, and cabbage will really expand when you put them into a food processor.

Chapter Thirteen

Questions

Most Frequently Asked Questions

Wherever I go, there seems to be a consistency to the questions that I am asked. The following is a compilation of your dieting and exercise questions, and the answers I have researched to the best of my ability.

What is lower in fat, margarine or butter?

Both margarine and butter contain 11 grams of fat per tablespoon. The difference is that the fat in margarine is mostly polyunsaturated, while the fat in butter is saturated. Eating a diet high in saturated fat increases the risk of heart disease and high blood pressure.

How can I prevent my child from developing an eating disorder?

If your child is a picky eater, lay off, and let her pick. Teach your child that people come in all shapes and sizes, and that remarks about weight are unacceptable. Make sure that you set a good example with your own eating habits.

How can I talk to my wife about her weight?

You don't need to talk to your wife about her problem. She already knows she's overweight. You need to get her moving without being obvious. Ask her to take a walk, or offer to cook a meal and make it low fat. Show her a lot of affection and support, and more than likely she will bring up the subject herself.

Is it true that lipstick contains calories?

Get ready to be shocked. The average woman consumes up to nine pounds of lipstick over the course of a lifetime.

How do I know if I need calcium supplements?

If you aren't getting enough calcium from foods, are a smoker, or are on the Pill, chances are that you do need a calcium supplement. It is best absorbed if taken in doses of 500 milligrams or less.

How do I stop my constant eating?

Chances are you're eating out of boredom rather than hunger. You need to find alternatives to eating, like a sport or a hobby. You might need to make some new friends to keep you busy. Eat often to keep your energy up, but not more than six times a day.

Is it better to eat before or after I exercise? I've heard that it is better to eat before so that you can work off the calories.

All experts agree that a calorie is a calorie no matter when you use it. They also concur that it's most important to eat when you're less likely to overeat. Also, some people feel shaky when they work out on an empty stomach, while others feel sluggish

154

working out on a full one. A pre-workout snack might be the best bet.

I enjoy appetisers, but most are so fattening. Are there any low-calorie choices on the menu?

Stay away from nachos, mozzarella cheese, and those blooming onions. Order a vegetable platter, shrimp cocktail, or best of all, portabello mushrooms.

> ### Is it true that celery actually contains negative calories?
>
> The truth is there's no such thing as negative calories, but celery is one of the lowest calorie foods you can eat, at only six calories a stalk.

Will eating meat prevent me from losing weight?

Meat has great nourishment value, but you need to limit your portions. Even the leanest cuts of meat still contain some fat.

Am I losing nutrients if I switch to skimmed milk?

Actually, quite the opposite. Skimmed milk is higher in calcium and protein than whole milk. The only downside is getting used to the flavour. Gradually adding it to your diet will help make it taste less "watery".

How can I tell if a food is fattening if there's no labelling?

You can tell by taking just a bite. If it coats your tongue, your teeth, the back of your mouth, or makes your lips feel slippery, it's probably high in fat.

How can I keep from feeling so deprived when I exercise?

You need to think of exercise as adding to whatever you like to do, rather than subtracting. For instance, if you like TV, buy a treadmill and watch it while you exercise.

Besides coffee, is there anything that I can do at work to get rid of that mid-afternoon slump?

Revive tired muscles and stimulate blood flow by placing a plastic water bottle on the floor. Take off your shoe and gently roll your foot over it from your heels to your toes. Repeat with the other foot. This reflexology technique will pep you right up!

Are there any foods that can give me more stamina?

Choose proteins for more long-term energy. Meats and low dairy products will take longer to digest.

Does salt really cause water retention?

Too much salt in the diet not only causes puffiness in the face and body, but it can lead to health troubles in later years.

Isn't a craving just telling me what my body needs?

If that was so, you'd be craving a lot more spinach and whole grains. Most of the time, a craving is just wishful thinking or a need for something comforting (comfort foods).

Are the "natural" diet pills sold in health food stores really safe?

Not if they contain ephedrine (ma-huang). Overdoses of this herb have been reported to cause rare cases of stroke, seizure, heart attack, and even death.

Is it true that toast has fewer calories than bread?

No, toasting bread, bagels, or other breads does nothing to alter its chemistry. The calorie content remains the same.

Why do plateaus occur in dieting?

Plateaus usually happen after a dieter has been dieting for some time. The real reason is that after some weight is lost, dieters need to drop their calorie allowance or increase their exercise even further to allow for further weight loss. Making this adjustment seems to get the weight moving again.

Is it possible to speed up metabolism?

The best way to increase metabolism is to increase muscle mass. Muscle requires more energy to maintain than fat. The more body fat, the harder it is to lose weight.

Is there any way to lose weight in a certain area of the body?

Unfortunately, there's no way to predict where weight will be lost. Spot reducing is a myth, and it's not even possible to spot reduce by exercising. There are certain body types that are earmarked by genetics.

How can I stay motivated throughout my diet?

Motivation seems to suffer when dieters make unrealistic goals and demands on their bodies. This results in discouragement and backsliding. Keep goals realistic, and allow for a few minor setbacks.

Should I stop working out if I'm sore?

Some soreness is natural when exercising. Usually getting moving again will make it feel better. If it doesn't stop in a day or two, cut back a little bit. However, if it's actually pain that you're experiencing, stop exercising. Ice the joint, and if it doesn't heal in a few days, see a doctor.

How do I get enough calcium in my diet if I don't eat dairy products?

There is calcium in dark green leafy vegetables. Unless you're eating five servings of these a day, you should take a calcium supplement.

Is sugar really bad for you?

Too much sugar in a diet is not conducive to weight loss because it's immediately turned into reserve fat. It's also a factor in diabetes and hardening of the arteries, often found in the obese.

Is there any difference in olive oil, peanut oil, sunflower oil, and safflower oil?

No, they all contain the same calories, about 120 per tablespoon.

> ### I know it's important to dring eight to ten glasses of water a day. Does diet soda count?
>
> Yes, as long as the soda is decaffeinated. Caffeine is a diuretic and can cause dehydration. The purpose of drinking fluids is to hydrate the body. However, diet soda can cause bloating, so water is still your best bet.

Is it nutritionally sound to occasionally substitute cereal for a meal?

Wholegrain, vitamin-fortified cereals with fruit are a great quick meal that can be substituted for lunch or dinner if the rest of the day's menu is balanced.

Does muscle really weigh more than fat?

Absolutely! A one-pound slab of fat weighs just one pound, obviously. However, that same amount of fat would weigh 22 per cent more as muscle, because muscle is more dense.

Is it true that you can eat certain foods in combination with other foods to burn calories more efficiently?

Every scientist and expert I questioned on this came up with same answer, NO! They tell me it makes absolutely no biological sense. Furthermore, it goes against all scientific knowledge of body chemistry and digestion.

Is it true that I increase my risk of diabetes if I'm overweight?

At least 80 per cent of people with diabetes were overweight at diagnosis. So it is true that maintaining a healthy weight will reduce the risk of developing diabetes. If you have diabetes, losing weight can help bring blood-sugar levels to more normal levels and reduce risk of diabetic complications.

What is the normal amount of weight gained just before menstruation?

According to most gynaecologists, the range of normal weight gain is from 1 to 4 pounds. Any more weight gained is due to dietary changes (PMS cravings).

> **What are good protein sources if I've decided to give up all meats including chicken and fish?**
>
> Low-fat dairy products, beans, rice, peanut butter, and tofu are all excellent replacements if you've decided to alter your diet in this manner.

How do I figure out how many calories a day to eat in order to lose weight?

You need to consume 15 calories per pound of body weight. No more than 30 per cent of those calories should come from fat. Realistically a good target calorie count is around 1200 calories on average. Any less is too difficult to maintain for a long period.

Can I still eat cheese and lose weight? I've heard that it's one of the worst foods for losing weight.

If you love cheese, and can't live without it, choose varieties that are softer in texture. Eating bread or fruit with the cheese will fill you up more quickly.

Do fruit juices contain any fibre?

They contain no fibre at all. Eat the fruit itself if you're looking for a good fibre source.

Is it all right to still include wine with my meals if I'm trying to drop a few pounds?

Yes, you can still have wine if you remember to count it as part of your meal. A good way to do this is to substitute a slice of bread, or take about 70 calories away from your meal.

What is a good low-fat treat to have after dinner?

Try a little diet jelly with a dollop of whipped cream on top, or eat a couple of marshmallows. Both these choices will set you back a mere 10 to 20 calories.

I can't watch a movie without munching on something. Any ideas?

A lot of dieters reported that instead of high-fat concession stand popcorn, they brought in a bag of cereal, like Kellogg's Corn Pops. These cereals provide that crunchy, sweet satisfaction without the fat.

What has more health advantages, stationary cycling or regular bicycling?

They provide equal health benefits, but the former can be truly boring unless you can read or watch a programme to make up for the loss of scenery.

How many different foods should I eat at a meal?

Dieters found that if they had too many choices at a meal, they were more likely to overeat. Giving yourself no more than three items at a time provided the right variety and nutrition.

Is there any way to trim down my favourite food, pizza?

If you order your pizza with a thin crust, and with little or no cheese, you can make a nutritious meal. Ask for extra vegetables like mushrooms and onions, and leave off the pepperoni. It contains too many calories.

What are the biggest dieting gimmicks around today?

Oh gee, where do I start? There's those patches that you apply to your skin that promise to melt fat while you sleep. Oh yes, and don't let me forget those creams and lotions that promise to reduce inches. There seems to be something new popping up every day. If it advertises "working overnight" or "melt fat in minutes" stay away. Hey, did you hear the one about the breath spray that curbs all your food cravings?

If I eat a cereal with raisins, how much do I need to equal a serving of fruit?

A normal one-ounce serving of cereal with raisins contains less than ¼ cup. It would take about three servings of cereal to get a full serving of fruit, so you'll need to add more raisins, or for a lower calorie count, blueberries.

I understand that potatoes are a good diet choice, but what size is a serving?

A small potato, about the size of your fist, or four inches long is about a serving.

Is it true that light mayonnaise is still high in fat?

Even light mayonnaise gets 75 per cent of its calories from fat. If it's mayo's slightly sour flavour you love, mix one cup of plain nonfat yoghurt with one tablespoon of mustard.

Chapter Fourteen

Recipes under 200 Calories

Enjoy Your Favourite Foods!

The recipes in this chapter are real food! These are recipes that you would be absolutely proud to serve your family and friends. I have also intentionally chosen recipes that are easy to make, with products that are readily available.

I encountered lots of difficulty while researching recipes for this chapter. Many recipes that were allegedly "slimming" were anywhere from 500 to 600 calories. That's not a diet recipe to me. Other recipes had as many as 20 to 25 ingredients. If you're like me, you would not attempt to cook with that many steps. Our lives are just too busy, and we're too hungry to wait! After the fifth ingredient, I'm out the door to the nearest fast food outlet. What you'll love about this chapter is that each of the recipes are a cinch to make, and absolutely delicious! Plus, you can mix and match until you get the number of calories you'd like to consume for any particular day.

I've tried to include something for everyone's taste. The last thing I would do is tell you to eat cauliflower if you hate it. There are also some low-fat desserts for those of us who just can't end a meal without a "little something" sweet. Trust me, your family will not know the desserts are low fat, and neither will your taste buds. Enjoy!

Appetizers and Dips under 200 Calories

Hot Spinach Artichoke Dip

95 calories per serving
Makes 24 servings

1 cup grated Parmesan cheese
1 cup low-fat mayonnaise
1 can (14 ounces) artichoke hearts, drained and chopped
1 package chopped spinach, thawed and drained
2 tablespoons tomato
Garlic, salt, and pepper to taste

Heat oven to 350 degrees. Mix all ingredients, except tomato. Spoon into 9-inch plate or quiche dish. Bake 30 to 35 minutes or until lightly browned. Serve topped with chopped tomato.

Stuffed Mushrooms

41 calories per serving
Makes 4 servings

12 large mushrooms
2 tablespoons lemon juice, divided
1 small red onion, chopped
1 teaspoon dill
2 tablespoons nonfat plain yoghurt
1 teaspoon mustard (preferably Dijon)
Salt and pepper to taste

Finely chop mushroom stems, leaving caps whole. Over high heat combine 1 tablespoon lemon juice with 2 pints of water. Bring to the boil. Add mushroom caps and cook until tender. Transfer to a bowl filled with iced water. Drain and pat dry. In a separate bowl, combine red onion, dill, yoghurt, mustard, and remaining lemon juice. Evenly divide filling among mushroom caps.

Salsa Dip

60 calories per serving
Makes 24 servings

1 pound processed cheese spread
1 eight-ounce jar salsa

Microwave cheese spread and salsa in a four-pint microwave proof bowl. Heat for 5 minutes on high. Stir after 3 minutes. Serve with baked tortilla chips, pepper wedges, or baked potato skins.

Pizza Potato Skins

65 calories per serving
Makes 24 servings

6 large baking potatoes
1 tablespoon oil
2 green peppers, diced
1 large onion, diced
2-ounce stick pepperoni, diced
¼ teaspoon salt
¼ teaspoon pepper
2 cans (8 ounces each) tomato sauce
2 tablespoons balsamic vinegar
2 ounces part-skimmed shredded mozzarella cheese

Preheat oven to 400 degrees. Bake potatoes until tender. In a skillet, heat oil and add peppers, onion, pepperoni, salt, and pepper. Cook until vegetables are soft. Stir in sauce and vinegar. Cook until thickened and set aside. Cut potatoes lengthwise and scoop out potato, leaving shell. Cut lengthwise again. Transfer to baking sheet. Divide sauce evenly over potato strips. Sprinkle each with cheese. Bake until cheese is melted and skins are crisp.

Portobello-Stuffed Courgette Boats

26 calories per serving
Makes 6 servings

3 medium courgettes, cut in half lengthwise
Olive oil nonstick cooking spray
2 portobello mushrooms, finely chopped
1 medium red pepper, finely chopped
1 tablespoon vinegar
3 tablespoons white wine

Preheat oven to 450 degrees. Scoop out insides of courgette. Chop courgette meat and set aside. Spray courgette skins with oil and bake 10 minutes. Meanwhile, cook mushroom, pepper, courgette meat, and vinegar in skillet over high heat. Add wine and cook until liquid is absorbed. Divide mixture among courgette skins. Bake until tops are slightly browned.

Southwestern Popcorn Mix

75 calories per serving
Makes 8 servings

6 cups air-popped popcorn
2 cups Cheerios cereal
2 tablespoons margarine
½ cup chilli powder
½ cup garlic powder
2 tablespoons grated Parmesan cheese

Mix popcorn and cereal in large bowl. Heat margarine with chilli and garlic powder until melted. Drizzle over mixture and toss until evenly coated. Sprinkle with cheese.

Black Bean and Corn Won Ton Cups

50 calories per serving

Makes 36 servings

36 won ton skins
1 cup chunky salsa
1 can whole kernel corn
1 can black beans, rinsed and drained
½ cup fat-free sour cream

Heat oven to 375 degrees. Line nonstick small muffin tins with won ton skins. Bake 10 minutes until golden. Remove from pan and cool. Mix remaining ingredients except sour cream. Spoon mixture evenly into cups. Top each with sour cream.

Hot Spinach Dip

55 calories per serving
Makes 20 servings

1 8-ounce package cream cheese
1 cup fat-free sour cream
2 tablespoons lemon juice
2 tablespoons Worcestershire sauce
2 tablespoons milk
1 teaspoon mustard powder
2 packages (10 ounces) frozen chopped spinach, thawed and drained
½ cup diced red peppers

Preheat oven to 375 degrees. Beat together cream cheese, sour cream, lemon juice, Worcestershire sauce, milk, and mustard powder until smooth. Gently stir in spinach and peppers. Bake in casserole dish until mixture bubbles around the edges. Serve with cut carrots, celery, etc.

Creamy Leek Dip

65 calories per serving

Makes 10 servings

2 cups low-fat small curd cottage cheese
¼ cup skimmed milk
1 packet leek soup mix
1 cup fresh parsley sprigs

In a food processor fitted with its metal blade, combine all ingredients except parsley sprigs until smooth. Add parsley and process until it is finely chopped. Place in a medium bowl and refrigerate for at least 2 hours.

Baked Onion Rings

51 calories per serving
Makes 4 servings

6 tablespoons seasoned dry breadcrumbs
½ large sweet yellow onion
1 egg white

Preheat oven to 450 degrees. Slice onion as thinly as possible. Separate into rings. Dip onion first in egg white, then in bread crumbs. Place on a nonstick baking sheet. Bake 10 minutes.

Crab Meat Spread

28 calories per serving
Makes 12 servings

1 cup crab meat
½ cup celery, diced
1 small onion, diced
½ green pepper, diced
1 cup sprouts
1 cup low-fat cottage cheese
Vinegar

Blend all above ingredients using enough vinegar to moisten. Season to taste.

Ham and Cheddar Bites

80 calories per serving
Makes 20 Servings

1 package (10 biscuits) refrigerated biscuit dough
3 tablespoons orange marmalade
¼ cup water
1 tablespoon orange juice
1 teaspoon apple cider vinegar
½ teaspoon cumin
4 ounces sliced ham cut into 20 pieces
2 ounces cheddar cheese sliced into 20 pieces

Preheat oven to 350 degrees. Cut each biscuit dough piece in half crosswise and place on a baking sheet. Bake 10 minutes or until golden. Heat water and marmalade in small pan. Add orange juice, vinegar, and cumin. Cook until mixture thickens. Assemble by topping each biscuit with ham and cheese. Then top with marmalade mix.

Soups under 200 Calories

Chilli Soup

175 calories per serving
Makes 5 servings

½ pound lean ground beef
1 tablespoon instant minced onion flakes
1 large can (16 ounces) red kidney beans, undrained
1 can (11 ounces) condensed reduced-fat tomato soup

1 soupcan water
3 teaspoons chilli powder

In a large pan, cook beef and onion over high heat until browned. Drain. Stir in remaining ingredients. Heat to boiling, stirring occasionally.

Egg Drop Soup

42 calories per serving
Makes 4 servings

2 cans (15 ounces) reduced-fat chicken stock
3 egg whites, slightly beaten
1 teaspoon soy sauce
¼ cup chopped scallions

In a medium saucepan, bring chicken stock to the boil. Cook uncovered for 5 minutes to reduce volume. Add egg whites and cook, stirring occasionally until white and stringy. Remove from heat and stir in soy sauce and scallions.

Gazpacho

52 calories per serving
Makes 6 servings

1 cucumber, peeled, cut, and seeded
2 ½ cups fresh tomatoes
1 large green pepper, chopped
1 large onion, chopped
1 teaspoon garlic flavoring
1 teaspoon dried chive
1 teaspoon paprika
Salt and pepper to taste
½ teaspoon sugar
2 cups tomato juice

2 tablespoons lemon juice

Shred cucumber with grater. Combine tomatoes, pepper, onion, garlic, chive, paprika, salt, and pepper. Add shredded cucumber to mixture. Stir in remaining ingredients. Cover and chill for at least 2 hours before serving.

Yellow Pepper and Orange Soup

35 calories per serving
Makes 4 servings

2 yellow bell peppers, halved and seeded
1 large onion, chopped
Grated rind and juice of 1 orange
1 ½ cups chicken stock
4 black olives, chopped
Salt and pepper to taste

Preheat oven to broil. Place peppers skin side up on baking sheet. Broil until skins are blackened. Cover and leave to cool. Place onion and orange juice in a small pan. Bring to the boil, then cover and simmer for 10 minutes. Peel peppers and blend with onion, half of the orange rind, and chicken stock. Season to taste, then heat gently. Serve sprinkled with olives and remaining rind.

Vichyssoise

149 calories per serving
Makes 6 servings

3 medium leeks
3 potatoes, peeled and diced
3 cups chicken broth
2 cups evaporated skimmed milk
Freshly ground pepper

Cut and discard roots and tough leaves from leeks. Cut leeks in half lengthwise and rinse under cold water. Then cut leeks crosswise, into ¼-inch-thick slices.

Spray a saucepan with cooking spray. Heat the pan over medium heat. Add leeks, potatoes, and broth, cooking and stirring for 5 minutes. Reduce heat and simmer for 30 minutes. Transfer leek mixture to food processor. Blend until smooth. Stir in milk and pepper. Soup may be chilled before serving.

Tortellini Soup

105 calories per serving
Makes 4 servings

3 cups beef broth
1 cup frozen cheese tortellini
1 cup frozen peas
2 tablespoons sun-dried tomatoes
1 teaspoon dried basil

In a medium saucepan, combine all ingredients. Cover and bring to the boil. Reduce heat and simmer for 5 minutes or until tortellini are tender.

Vegetable Soup

75 calories per serving
Makes 8 servings

16 ounces tomato juice
16 ounces water
14 ounces chicken broth
16 ounces peeled tomatoes
½ pound green beans, cut into 1-inch pieces
¾ pound carrots, sliced
3 celery stalks, sliced

1 onion, sliced
1 courgette, sliced
1 summer squash, sliced

Combine tomato juice, water, broth, and tomatoes. Bring to the boil. Add remaining ingredients. Bring to the boil and simmer for 30 minutes. Season to taste.

Mixed Bean Soup

95 calories a serving
Makes 4 servings

1 teaspoon olive oil
1 red onion, chopped
1 garlic clove, crushed
⅔ cup tomato paste
1 teaspoon dried thyme
1 ½ cups frozen or fresh green beans
15-ounce can cannelloni beans
Salt and pepper to taste

Heat the olive oil in a pan, then sauté onion and garlic until tender but not brown. Add the tomato paste and thyme and bring to the boil. Add the green beans, cover and simmer for about 6 minutes or until tender. Add beans and season to taste.

Salads under 200 Calories

One-Minute Chicken Salad

160 calories per serving
Makes 1 serving

5-ounce can premium chicken breast in water
2 tablespoons light mayonnaise
1 cup celery, diced
1 tablespoon finely diced onion

Drain chicken. Mix with mayonnaise, celery, and onion.

Greek Salad

90 calories per serving
Makes 2 servings

2 cups romaine lettuce
2 tablespoons feta cheese
1 tomato
1 cucumber
½ stalk celery, sliced
2 black olives
2 tablespoons vinegar
1 tablespoon olive oil

Toss all ingredients together and serve.

Fresh Pea Salad

70 calories per serving
Makes 12 servings

4 cups fresh peas
3 tablespoons fresh chive, chopped
2 tablespoons wine vinegar

2 tablespoons olive oil
½ teaspoon salt
2 red peppers, chopped
1 head Boston lettuce, thinly sliced

Over medium heat, bring peas and enough salted water to cover to the boil. Cook until tender. Rinse under cold water and drain. Whisk together chive, vinegar, oil, and salt. Add peas, peppers, and lettuce. Toss well to coat.

Citrus Salad

160 calories per serving
Makes 4 servings

2 seedless oranges
1 grapefruit
1 tablespoon honey
1 tablespoon olive oil
1 tablespoon balsamic vinegar
6 cups torn mixed greens
1 small red onion, sliced
Salt and pepper to taste

Peel oranges and grapefruit. Cut into 1/4-inch slices, then quarters. Combine olive oil, honey, and vinegar. Toss greens with dressing and red onion. Add orange and grapefruit pieces.

Noodle Salad

120 calories per serving
Makes 6 servings

8 ounces thin spaghetti
1 red pepper, sliced into thin strips
1 small cucumber, cut into thin strips
½ cup carrot, grated

2 green onions, thinly sliced
2 tablespoons rice vinegar
2 tablespoons teriyaki
2 tablespoons water
1 tablespoon soy sauce
1 teaspoon sesame oil

Cook spaghetti until just tender. Drain and rinse in cold water and transfer to large bowl. Add red pepper, cucumber, carrot, and onions, and mix well. In a small bowl, mix vinegar, teriyaki, water, soy sauce, and sesame oil. Pour sauce over noodle mix.

German Potato Salad

180 calories per serving
Makes 4 servings

1 ½ pounds small red potatoes
3 shallots or leeks, minced
¼ cup each of parsley, chive, and thyme
2 tablespoons balsamic or wine vinegar
2 tablespoons beef broth
2 tablespoons olive oil
2 garlic cloves, minced

Boil potatoes in saucepan until tender. Remove from heat, drain, and cut in halves. In a medium bowl, toss with shallots or leeks. Toss in parsley, chive, and thyme and set aside. In a small saucepan, combine vinegar, beef broth, olive oil, and garlic. Warm over low heat and pour over potatoes. Fold in carefully before serving.

Red Coleslaw

40 calories per serving
Makes 4 servings

½ small red cabbage, shredded
1 red onion, thinly sliced
4 radishes, thinly sliced
1 red apple, cored and grated
1 tablespoon low-fat plain yoghurt
1 teaspoon honey
Salt and pepper to taste

Place cabbage, onion, radishes, and apple in salad bowl. Toss. In a screw-top jar, shake the yoghurt, honey, salt, and pepper until they are blended. Pour the dressing over the salad. Toss and serve.

Couscous Salad

105 calories per serving
Makes 4 servings

1 ½ cups couscous
1 celery stalk, chopped
½ small cauliflower, cut into small florets
4 scallions, chopped
3 tablespoons dried parsley
1 tablespoon lemon juice
½ teaspoon chilli sauce
Salt and pepper to taste

Cook couscous according to package directions. Leave to cool. Stir in remaining ingredients. Season and toss. Spoon on to a large platter and serve.

Deli Salad

180 calories per serving
Makes 8 servings

7-ounce can of artichoke hearts, drained
1 cup cubed mozzarella cheese

1 cup rotini pasta, cooked and drained
2 ½-ounce cans pitted olives
½ cup low-fat Italian dressing
1 cup red onion rings
½ cup green pepper, chopped
¼ cup Parmesan cheese, shredded

Mix all ingredients together. Refrigerate before serving.

Spinach Salad

80 calories per serving
Makes 4 servings

2 cups fresh spinach
½ cup dried apricots, chopped
2 tablespoons sunflower seeds
1 tablespoon sesame seeds
2 tablespoons orange juice
1 tablespoon balsamic vinegar
2 tablespoons low-fat plain yoghurt
Salt and pepper to taste

Tear up spinach and place in large bowl. Add apricots, sunflower seeds, and sesame seeds. In a small bowl, mix together orange juice, vinegar, and yoghurt. Pour over spinach mixture. Add salt and pepper. Refrigerate before serving.

Waldorf Salad

60 calories per serving
Makes 10 servings

6 cups apples, diced
2 ½ cups celery, thinly sliced
½ cup raisins
½ cup nonfat mayonnaise

¼ cup nonfat sour cream

Combine apples, celery, and raisins in a large bowl. Stir to mix well. In a small bowl, combine mayonnaise with sour cream. Stir. Add mayonnaise mixture to apple mixture and toss together. Refrigerate for 2 hours before serving.

Chicken and Pasta Salad

165 calories per serving
Makes 8 servings

3 cups chicken broth
1 pound boneless chicken breasts
2 cups shell pasta
1 cup nonfat mayonnaise
1 teaspoon mustard
½ teaspoon celery salt
Ground pepper to taste
2 ribs of celery, thinly sliced
1 cup baby peas, cooked, drained, and cooled
1 cup seedless red grapes, washed and cut in half

Bring chicken broth to a simmer in medium saucepan. Add chicken breasts and cook for 20 minutes. Remove breasts and chill. Cook pasta according to directions, drain, and rinse in cold water. Mix together mayonnaise, mustard, celery salt, and pepper. Cut chicken into bite-size pieces and add to mixture. Add pasta, celery, peas, and grapes. Toss together. Cover and refrigerate for one hour.

Arugula and Orange Salad

50 calories per serving
Makes 6 servings

1 bunch arugula, stems removed
9 radishes, thinly sliced

1 red onion, thinly sliced
1 orange, peeled and sectioned
1 tablespoon chicken broth
Juice and grated zest of 1 lime
1 clove garlic, minced
½ teaspoon ground cumin
½ teaspoon salt
1 teaspoon olive oil

Combine arugula, radishes, onion, and orange sections. In separate bowl combine chicken broth, lime juice and zest, garlic, cumin, and salt. Whisk in oil until mixture thickens slightly. Add to salad.

Cucumber Salad with Dill

50 calories per serving
Makes 4 servings

2 cucumbers
3 tablespoons vinegar
1 tablespoon sugar
Salt and pepper to taste
1 red onion, sliced and made into rings
1 teaspoon dried dill weed

Wash the cucumbers and partially remove peel in lengthwise strips. Use a fork to leave a little skin between each strip and slice crosswise. Combine vinegar, sugar, salt, and pepper in a bowl until sugar is dissolved. Add cucumber, onion, and dill. Toss well. Serve immediately.

Vegetable Salad

55 calories per serving
Makes 8 servings

3 cups broccoli, chopped

3 cups cauliflower, chopped
1 cup celery, sliced
20 black olives, pitted and sliced
15-ounce can mushrooms, drained
¾ cup fat-free Italian salad dressing

Combine all ingredients in a large bowl. Stir to cover vegetables. Chill for at least 3 hours before serving.

Low-Fat Salad Dressings

Creamy Ranch Dressing

15 calories per tablespoon
Makes 1 cup

¾ cup plain nonfat yoghurt
¼ cup low-fat mayonnaise
1 tablespoon cider vinegar
2 teaspoons Dijon mustard
¼ teaspoon dried thyme
1 green onion, minced

Mix all ingredients together. Cover and refrigerate. Stir before serving.

Creamy Italian Dressing

10 calories per tablespoon
Makes 1 cup

½ cup fat-free sour cream
⅓ cup nonfat buttermilk
2 tablespoons grated Parmesan cheese
1 teaspoon dried basil, crushed
1 clove garlic, minced
Salt and pepper to taste

Mix the sour cream and buttermilk in a small bowl until smooth. Stir in Parmesan, basil, garlic, salt, and pepper. Refrigerate.

Vegetable Dishes under 200 Calories

Snow Peas and Carrots

80 calories per serving
Makes 4 servings

1 onion, thinly sliced
4 teaspoons olive oil
2 carrots, cut into 2-inch strips
½ pound snow peas, strings removed
2 teaspoons dried dill
Salt and pepper to taste

Microwave onion and oil for 1 minute. Stir in carrots, cover with plastic, and microwave for 2 minutes. Stir in snow peas and dill. Microwave covered for 6 minutes. Let stand for 3 minutes. Season and serve.

Carrots and Grapes

45 calories per serving
Makes 4 servings

2 cups carrots, sliced
1 shallot, chopped
¼ cup water
2 tablespoons red wine vinegar
1 tablespoon brown sugar
½ cup seedless grapes, halved

In nonstick skillet, cook carrots and shallot in water for about 10 minutes. Stir until carrots are tender. Push carrot mixture to side of skillet. Stir in vinegar and sugar. Gently add in grapes. Toss all together.

Hash Browns

96 calories per serving
Makes 4 servings

4 medium-size potatoes
1 onion
Nonfat cooking spray
Paprika

Preheat oven to 400 degrees. Cut potatoes into cubes. Cut onion into small pieces. Spray 9 x 9-inch pan with cooking spray. Place cut potatoes and onion in pan. Sprinkle with a little water, then sprinkle with paprika. Bake for 20 minutes, then remove from oven. Heat oven to broiling, then cook mixture until potatoes are brown.

Courgette Frittata

65 calories per serving
Makes 4 servings

2 small courgettes
1 teaspoon water
2 green onions, chopped
1 teaspoon basil
1 teaspoon dried marjoram
1 ½ cups egg substitute
2 tablespoons Parmesan cheese

Cut each courgette lengthwise into quarters. Thinly slice each quarter. Place the water in a 10-inch skillet. Add courgettes and onions. Cook over low heat for about 3 minutes. Discard cooking liquid. Stir in basil and marjoram. Carefully pour egg substitute over courgettes and onions. Cook over low heat until mixture starts

Vegetable Dishes

to set. Lift edges of uncooked mixture to flow underneath. Continue cooking until nearly set. Sprinkle with cheese. Broil for 1 minute and serve.

Peas and Onions

105 calories per serving
Makes 8 servings

16-ounce package frozen small whole onions
2 tablespoons butter
20 ounces frozen peas, thawed
2 tablespoons chopped mint
1 tablespoon Parmesan cheese
Salt and pepper to taste

Cook onions according to package directions. Drain. Melt butter in skillet and add onions and peas cooking for 3 minutes. Place in bowl, toss with mint, cheese, salt, and pepper.

Rosemary "Fries"

75 calories per serving
Makes 4 servings

3 large baking potatoes
2 teaspoons olive oil
1 teaspoon rosemary
Salt and pepper to taste

Preheat broiler. Cut potatoes lengthwise into 3 slices each. Cut each slice into 3 large French fries. Cook potatoes in microwave with a bit of water. Take out while still crisp (not mashing soft). Spread steamed potatoes on baking sheet sprayed with cooking spray. Sprinkle with olive oil and dried rosemary. Broil until potatoes are golden brown. Turn and brown other side. Season and serve.

Sesame Broccoli and Cauliflower

50 calories per serving
Makes 1 serving

¼ cup cauliflower florets
¾ cup broccoli
½ teaspoon soy sauce
¼ teaspoon sesame oil
Salt and pepper to taste

Combine soy sauce, sesame oil, salt, and pepper in microwave-proof bowl. Add broccoli and cauliflower. Cover and microwave on high for 1 minute. Uncover and toss.

Orange-Glazed Asparagus

45 calories per serving
Makes 8 servings

2 tablespoons butter
2 packs (10 ounces each) frozen asparagus
¼ cup orange juice
¼ cup white wine
1 teaspoon orange peel
Salt and pepper to taste

In large skillet, melt butter over medium heat. Add asparagus and cook until heated through. Transfer to a dish. In same skillet, add orange juice, wine, peel, salt, and pepper. Cook until reduced by half. Pour over asparagus.

Glazed Carrots

70 calories per serving
Makes 4 servings

1 pound carrots
1 cup water
4 teaspoons apple juice
1 tablespoon brown sugar
1 teaspoon butter
½ teaspoon nutmeg

Cut carrots into 2-inch pieces, then quarter them lengthwise. Microwave carrots for 5 minutes until just tender. Meanwhile, stir together water, apple juice, brown sugar, and butter. Microwave for 30 seconds or until sugar and butter just melt. Drizzle carrots with juice mixture. Toss to coat. Serve sprinkled with nutmeg.

Rice Almondine

115 calories per serving
Makes 6 servings

1 cup onion, chopped
1 ¼ cups chicken broth
1 tablespoon lemon juice
½ teaspoon garlic powder
1 ½ cups minute brown rice
1 cup frozen green beans, thawed
2 tablespoons toasted slivered almonds
½ teaspoon dried dill weed.

Coat medium saucepan with cooking spray. Add onion and cook until tender. Add chicken broth, lemon juice, and garlic powder. Bring to the boil. Stir in rice and return to the boil. Reduce heat to low. Cover and simmer for about 5 minutes. Remove from heat and stir in remaining ingredients. Fluff with fork and serve.

Swiss Asparagus Au Gratin

170 calories per serving
Makes 4 servings

½ cup water
1 ½ pounds asparagus spears, trimmed
½ cup Swiss cheese, shredded
¼ cup breadcrumbs
2 tablespoons butter, melted
½ teaspoon dry mustard
¼ teaspoon fresh ground pepper

Heat oven to 400 degrees. Bring 1/2 cup water to the boil in 10-inch skillet. Add asparagus. Cook for 2 minutes and drain. Place in 10 x 6-inch baking pan. Mix remaining ingredients. Sprinkle over asparagus. Bake for 10 minutes until cheese mixture is lightly browned.

Entrees under 200 Calories

Beef Tenderloin with Onions

175 calories per serving
Makes 4 servings

½ cup chicken broth
2 large onions, thinly sliced
4 cloves garlic, finely chopped
¼ cup balsamic vinegar
½ teaspoon salt
¼ teaspoon ground pepper
4 beef tenderloin steaks (totalling 1 pound)

Heat chicken broth to boiling in a 2-pint saucepan. Stir in onions and garlic. Cover and cook over medium heat until onions are soft. Stir in vinegar and cook uncovered until liquid has evaporated. Sprinkle beef with salt and pepper. Cook beef in nonstick skillet until desired doneness. Serve with onions.

Broiled Flank Steak

170 calories per serving
Makes 4 servings

1 pound lean flank steak
¾ cup dry red wine
3 garlic cloves, cut into quarters
1 bay leaf, cut in half
1 teaspoon onion powder
2 teaspoons Dijon mustard

Marinate steak in a baking dish with wine, garlic, and bay leaf for 1 hour. Preheat broiler. Drain steak. Place steak on a broiler rack. Sprinkle with onion powder. Spread a thin layer of mustard over the top. Broil to desired doneness.

Pineapple Steak Kebabs

185 calories per serving
Makes 4 servings

1 tablespoon soy sauce
2 tablespoons water
1 teaspoon garlic powder
1 tablespoon apple sauce
1 pound steak, cut into 2-inch squares
Small red bell pepper, cut into 1-inch squares
8-ounce can unsweetened pineapple chunks, juice reserved
8 fresh mushrooms

Combine soy sauce, water, garlic powder, and apple sauce.

Marinate over steak for 1 hour. Thread steak, pepper, pineapple, and mushrooms on skewers. Broil until desired doneness.

Meat Loaf

150 calories per serving
Makes 4 servings

¾ pound lean ground beef
¾ pound ground turkey breast
½ cup old-fashioned oatmeal
½ cup tomato puree
1 teaspoon Italian seasoning
½ teaspoon salt
1 small onion, chopped
1 clove garlic, finely chopped

Preheat oven to 375 degrees. Mix all ingredients thoroughly. Press mixture into ungreased loaf tin. Bake for about one hour or until centre is no longer pink.

Pork Steaks with Peppercorn Glaze

175 calories per serving
Makes 4 servings

4 lean pork loin steaks
1 tablespoon green peppercorns, crushed
4 tablespoons balsamic vinegar
½ cup chicken broth
4 scallions, sliced

Mix together peppercorns and vinegar. Sprinkle over pork. Marinate for 30 minutes. Reserving the peppercorn mixture, fry the pork in a nonstick pan. Add the peppercorn mix, broth, and scallions. Boil rapidly, uncovered, for about 10 minutes.

Lemon Chicken

130 calories per serving
Makes 4 servings

1 pound boneless chicken breast halves (4 pieces)
2 lemons
1 teaspoon dried tarragon
Fresh pepper to taste

Preheat oven to 350 degrees. Place chicken in foil-lined baking pan. Fold sides of the foil up. Halve lemons and squeeze juice of ½ lemon over each chicken piece. Sprinkle each piece with ¼ teaspoon tarragon and pepper to taste. Fold foil together and seal to secure chicken. Bake for about 45 minutes.

Feta and Mint Chicken Breasts

160 calories per serving
Makes 4 servings

4 6-ounce boneless, skinless chicken breast halves
1 ounce feta cheese, thinly sliced
1 cup fresh mint leaves
2 teaspoons olive oil
1 tablespoon lemon juice
Salt and pepper to taste

Pressing each breast, cut a pocket. Insert feta cheese and half of mint leaves evenly into each breast. Place breasts in baking dish. Finely chop remaining mint and add olive oil, lemon juice, salt, and pepper. Marinate for 30 minutes. Preheat broiler. Broil for 4 to 6 minutes per side.

Mediterranean Turkey Spirals

125 calories per serving
Makes 4 servings

4 thin turkey breast steaks
2 tablespoons pesto
½ cup basil leaves
½ cup chicken broth
½ cup tomato juice
Garlic, salt, and pepper to taste

Pound turkey until thin. Spread with pesto sauce. Lay basil leaves over each steak, then roll in a jelly roll fashion. Secure with toothpicks. Combine chicken broth and tomato juice. Bring to the boil over high heat. Add the turkey spirals, cover, and simmer for 15 minutes. Season, and remove toothpicks. Serve hot.

Turkey Meat Loaf

175 calories per serving
Makes 8 servings

1 ½ pounds ground turkey breast
½ cup seasoned breadcrumbs
½ cup uncooked oatmeal
½ cup low-fat milk
2 tablespoons soy sauce
1 large onion, chopped
1 egg
Fresh ground pepper

Preheat oven to 350 degrees. Mix all ingredients. Place mixture in a loaf pan coated with cooking spray. Bake for about 1 hour. Meat should not have any pink colour when done.

Tuna with Tomato Vinaigrette

110 calories per serving
Makes 6 servings

1 ½ cups water
½ cup sun-dried tomatoes
2 cloves garlic, sliced
¼ cup olive oil
¼ cup lemon juice
1 tablespoon dried thyme
6 tuna steaks (about 6 ounces each)
Salt and pepper to taste

Preheat broiler. Over medium heat, bring 1 ½ cups water to the boil. Add sun-dried tomatoes and cook until softened. Drain and reserve liquid. Cook garlic in olive oil until golden. Stir in tomatoes, lemon juice, thyme, and reserved liquid and leave simmering. Separately, sprinkle tuna with salt and pepper and broil until done. Top with simmering sauce.

Baked Scallops

125 calories per serving
Makes 4 servings

1 tablespoon butter
¼ cup white wine
Juice from one lemon
1 pound scallops

Preheat oven to 450 degrees. Heat all but the scallops in oven for 10 minutes. Pour liquid over scallops. Marinate in 9-inch casserole dish for 20 minutes at room temperature. Bake for about 15 minutes. Do not overcook.

Oysters Rockefeller

90 calories per serving
Makes 4 servings

2 teaspoons olive oil

1 tablespoon onion, grated
2 tablespoons breadcrumbs
Tarragon, pepper, and Tabasco to taste
10 ounces frozen chopped spinach, thawed and drained
8 ounces oysters, raw or canned
2 tablespoons mozzarella cheese, grated
1 tablespoon Parmesan cheese

Preheat broiler. Combine oil, onion, breadcrumbs, and seasoning. Toss mixture with spinach. Broil oysters for 5 to 7 minutes if using raw oysters. Drain liquid if using canned oysters. Top oysters with spinach mixture and broil for about 4 minutes. Sprinkle with cheeses and broil until just melted.

Devilled Shrimp

140 calories per serving
Makes 1 serving

5 jumbo shrimp, uncooked, peeled, and de-veined
2 tablespoons white wine
1 tablespoon Dijon mustard
1 garlic clove, crushed
¼ cup onions, diced
Salt and pepper to taste
1 tomato, peeled
¼ cup parsley, chopped

Coat skillet with cooking spray. Add shrimp and cook on high heat for about 2 minutes on each side. Add wine, mustard, garlic, onion, and seasonings. Cover and cook for about 8 minutes. Add tomato, breaking it up with a fork. Mix all together, cover again, and cook for 10 minutes. Add parsley and serve.

Seafood Bisque

130 calories per serving
Makes 8 servings

2 ½ cups frozen corn, thawed
2 cups chicken broth
1 tablespoon butter
2 green peppers, chopped
Salt and pepper to taste
1 cup low-fat milk
½ pound shrimp, peeled and de-veined
½ pound scallops
3 tablespoons parsley

In food processor, combine 2 cups of corn with 1 cup chicken broth. Purée until smooth. Melt butter over medium heat in a saucepan. Add peppers, onions, salt, and pepper to taste. Cook for 5 minutes. Stir in corn mixture, milk, and remaining broth. Cover and simmer for 5 minutes. Add shrimp, scallops, remaining corn, and parsley. Cook for about 5 minutes and serve.

Stir-Fried Tofu with Vegetables

150 calories per serving
Makes 4 servings

2 teaspoons vegetable oil
1 package (16 ounces) extra-firm tofu, patted dry and cut into 1-inch pieces
1 cup vegetable broth
1 tablespoon soy sauce
2 teaspoons flour
3 green onions, thinly sliced
1 bag (10 ounces) shredded carrots
1 medium red pepper, thinly sliced
2 garlic cloves, crushed in garlic press

1 tablespoon ginger
½ teaspoon salt

In a skillet, heat 1 teaspoon vegetable oil until hot, then add tofu. Cook for 4 minutes until golden. Transfer to plate and set aside. In a separate bowl, mix vegetable broth, soy sauce, and flour. In the same skillet, heat remaining teaspoon oil, white parts of green onions, carrots, pepper, garlic, ginger, and salt. Cook for 5 minutes, stirring frequently. Return tofu to skillet and stir in broth mixture. Heat to boiling and serve.

Baked Aubergine, Tomatoes, and Feta

95 calories per serving
Makes 4 servings

1 medium aubergine, thinly sliced
Garlic salt to taste
2 large tomatoes, sliced
1 cup feta cheese, crumbled
4 tablespoons plain yoghurt
Paprika to taste

Preheat oven to 400 degrees. Sprinkle the aubergine slices with garlic salt, leave for 30 minutes, then wipe salt off. Spray baking dish with cooking spray. Arrange aubergine and tomatoes to slightly overlap. Sprinkle with feta cheese and spoon over yoghurt. Sprinkle with paprika and garlic salt. Bake for 30 minutes or until bubbling and golden.

Vegetable Tortillas

180 calories per serving
Makes 6 servings

½ cup red pepper, diced
½ cup yellow pepper, diced

½ cup courgettes, diced
6 flour tortillas
1 ½ cups reduced-fat Monterey Jack cheese, shredded

Mix peppers and courgettes. Spoon ¼ cup of vegetable mixture on to centre of each tortilla. Top each with ¼ cup cheese. Roll tortilla tightly around mixture. Spray 10-inch skillet with nonstick cooking spray. Cook 3 tortillas seam side down until bottoms are light brown. Spray tops and turn. Cook for 3 minutes longer until brown. Repeat with remaining tortillas.

Enchiladas

160 calories per serving
Makes 6 servings

2 cups chunky salsa
Vegetable cooking spray
1 red bell pepper, thinly sliced
½ cup onion, thinly sliced
2 cups mushrooms, sliced
1 small potato, cut into 1/2-inch pieces
1 clove garlic, minced
¼ cup water
2 cups fresh spinach leaves, washed and dried
¼ teaspoon hot red pepper flakes
½ cup feta cheese, crumbled
6 corn tortillas
8 cups Romaine lettuce, finely shredded

Preheat oven to 375 degrees. Lightly spray 10-inch nonstick skillet with cooking spray. Add pepper and onion and cook until softened. Add mushrooms, potato, garlic, and ¼ cup water and cook until softened. Remove from heat and stir in spinach and pepper flakes until spinach is wilted. Add feta and stir to blend. Warm tortillas in skillet, about a minute each side. Place ⅓ cup of vegetable mixture in tortilla and roll up. Lightly spray square baking pan and place tortillas seam side down. Brush lightly with a little liquid from salsa. Cover with foil and bake for 20 minutes. Divide lettuce among 6 plates and place enchiladas on top. Top with salsa.

Vegetarian Stuffed Peppers

145 calories per serving
Makes 6 servings

6 green peppers
2 cups cooked rice
1 cup couscous
3 egg whites
Salt, pepper, and parsley to taste
¼ cup seasoned breadcrumbs
1 cup water
1 small onion, chopped
½ cup celery, chopped
8-ounce can tomato sauce

Preheat oven to 375 degrees. Cut peppers in half and remove seeds. Microwave for 2 minutes. Combine rice, cooked couscous, egg whites, and seasonings. Sprinkle in breadcrumbs and set aside as stuffing. Bring 1 cup of water to the boil. Add onion and celery, boil for 15 more minutes. Add tomato sauce, mix, and cook 20 minutes. Spray a baking dish with cooking spray. Fill peppers with stuffing. Cover with sauce. Bake for 40 minutes.

Pasta Primavera

180 calories per serving
Makes 4 servings

8 ounces uncooked linguine

1 cup green beans, in 1-inch pieces
1 medium carrot, cut into ¼-inch slices
½ medium green pepper
1 cup mushrooms, sliced
1 medium tomato, cut into 1-inch pieces
8-ounce bottle fat-free creamy Italian dressing

Cook linguine until tender, adding green beans, carrot, and pepper during last 5 minutes. While linguine is cooking, place mushrooms in colander. Drain linguine and vegetables in colander. Place linguine mixture in saucepan, adding in tomato and dressing. Cook over medium heat until hot.

Breads, Pizza, and Quiche under 200 Calories

Lemon Pepper Popovers

105 calories per serving
Makes 6 servings

1 cup flour
1 cup skimmed milk at room temperature
1 tablespoon olive oil
Salt and pepper to taste
2 teaspoons lemon zest
3 egg whites, slightly beaten

Preheat oven to 450 degrees. Mix together flour and milk. Add remaining ingredients, just enough to mix. Grease muffin cups with cooking spray. Fill each cup half full. Bake 15 minutes at 450 degrees. Reduce heat to 350 degrees for 20 more minutes. Serve at once.

Blueberry Muffins

123 calories per serving

Makes 12 muffins

2 cups flour
1 tablespoon baking powder
½ teaspoon salt
1 cup blueberries
4 egg whites
1 ½ cups nonfat yoghurt
½ cup sugar
1 teaspoon vanilla extract

Preheat oven to 400 degrees. Mix together flour, baking powder, and salt. Add blueberries. Stir lightly to coat and set aside. Beat egg whites to peaks. Add yoghurt, sugar, and vanilla. Add liquid mixture to dry ingredients and fold together gently. Place in non-stick 12-cup muffin tin. Optional: Place 1 blueberry in the center of each muffin. Sprinkle a little sugar over each muffin. Bake for 20 minutes.

Spiced Carrot Bread

125 calories per serving
Makes one loaf or 12 slices

2 eggs
4 tablespoons vegetable oil
3 tablespoons sugar
3 carrots, coarsely grated
1 ⅓ cups flour
1 teaspoon baking powder
2 teaspoons allspice
3 tablespoons skimmed milk

Preheat oven to 350 degrees. Line loaf pan with wax paper. Mix together eggs, oil, and sugar. Stir in carrots. Add flour, baking powder, and allspice. Fold in milk. Pour into pan. Bake 40 to 45 minutes.

Pizza Bread

135 calories per serving
Makes 6 servings

1 ½ cups flour
1 ½ teaspoons baking powder
½ teaspoon salt
¾ cup beer
½ cup spaghetti sauce
⅓ cup low-fat mozzarella cheese, shredded

Heat oven to 400 degrees. Spray round cake pan with nonstick cooking spray. Mix flour, baking powder, and salt in mixing bowl. Thoroughly stir in beer. Spread dough in pan and spread sauce over it. Bake for 15 minutes or until toothpick inserted in centre comes out clean.

Spicy Onion Tart

175 calories per serving
Makes 8 servings

1 tablespoon butter
4 large yellow onions, thinly sliced
1 cup nonfat sour cream
3 eggs
Salt, black pepper, and cayenne pepper to taste
One frozen pie shell
1 teaspoon dried parsley

Preheat oven to 375 degrees. Melt butter in large nonstick skillet. Add onions. Cover and cook for 15 minutes. Uncover and cook until browned. Remove from heat and let cool. Combine sour cream, eggs, peppers, and salt. Add onions. Pour into pie shell. Sprinkle with parsley. Bake for 30 to 35 minutes. Cool slightly before slicing.

Onion Twists

120 calories per serving
Makes 12 servings

1 large onion, thinly sliced
2 tablespoons olive oil
2 tablespoons parsley, minced
½ teaspoon coarse salt
1 pound frozen pizza dough, thawed
1 egg, beaten

Preheat oven to 400 degrees. Heat oil in skillet and cook onion over medium heat until golden. Stir in parsley and ¼ teaspoon salt. Roll dough out on floured surface to about 15 x 12-inches. Spread onion on lower half of dough, leaving a border. Fold dough lengthwise, seal, and brush with egg. Cut crosswise into 12 strips. Twist and place on nonstick baking pan. Brush with egg and sprinkle with remaining egg and salt. Bake until golden.

Broiled Crisp Bread

100 calories per serving
Makes 12 servings

2 cups flour
1 teaspoon salt
4 tablespoons butter, melted
½ cup warm water
1 teaspoon red pepper flakes
Salt and pepper to taste

Preheat broiler. Combine flour and salt. Stir in 2 tablespoons butter. Stir in water 1 tablespoon at a time. Divide dough into 12 pieces and roll each piece into a circle. Coat baking pan with cooking spray. Broil circles for 2 minutes on each side, brushing with butter. Sprinkle with salt, pepper, and flakes. Broil one more minute.

Desserts under 200 Calories

Lemon Bars

150 calories per serving
Makes 24 bars

1 cup shortening
1 cup brown sugar
1 ½ cups flour
1 teaspoon baking powder
1 teaspoon cinnamon
1 cup quick-cooking oats
8 ounces light cream cheese, softened
½ cup sugar
½ cup lemon juice
2 teaspoons grated lemon peel

Preheat oven to 350 degrees. Beat together shortening and brown sugar. Add flour, baking powder, and cinnamon. Stir in oats. Reserve 1½ cups oat mixture. Press remaining oat mixture on to bottom of greased 13 x 9-inch pan. Beat cream cheese with sugar, juice, and peel. Pour over oat mixture. Sprinkle with remaining mixture. Bake for about 30 minutes.

Apple Crisp

135 calories per serving
Makes 8 servings

4 apples, sliced
⅓ cup brown sugar
¼ cup flour
¼ cup rolled oats
1 teaspoon cinnamon
2 tablespoons butter, softened

Preheat oven to 375 degrees. Coat an 8 x 8-inch pan with cooking spray. Place apple slices in pan. Mix remaining ingredients together. Sprinkle over apples. Bake 30 minutes.

Apple Nut Cookies

75 calories per serving
Makes 14 cookies

1 ½ cups rolled oats
1 teaspoon allspice
4 tablespoons shortening
3 tablespoons brown sugar
1 apple, cored and chopped
3 tablespoons walnuts
1 egg white

Preheat oven to 400 degrees. Mix together oats, allspice, and shortening. Add brown sugar, apple, walnuts, and egg white. Stir. Form 14 balls. Arrange on nonstick baking pan. Flatten slightly. Bake for 10 minutes.

Chocolate Truffles

60 calories per serving
Makes about 30 truffles

½ cup chopped raisins
2 tablespoons chocolate-flavoured liqueur
40 squares graham crackers ground to a powder
14-ounce can sweetened condensed skimmed milk
½ cup unsweetened cocoa powder
1 teaspoon vanilla

Combine raisins and liqueur. Let stand until softened. Combine crackers, milk, ¼ cup cocoa powder, vanilla, and raisin mixture. Chill one hour. Place remaining cocoa powder in shallow bowl. Shape chocolate mixture into balls. Roll in cocoa powder. Freeze 15 minutes. Store in refrigerator.

Biscotti

65 calories per serving
Makes 24 servings

3 cups flour
1 teaspoon baking powder
5 tablespoons shortening
⅔ cup sugar
3 eggs
1 tablespoon lemon juice
1 cup currants
¾ cup dried apricots

Preheat oven to 350 degrees. Combine flour and baking powder. Set aside. Cream together shortening and sugar. Beat in eggs. Add lemon juice. Add dry ingredients. Add currants and apricots. Divide and shape dough into 2 loaves. Bake for 30 minutes.

Cheesecake Cups

129 calories per serving
Makes 8 servings

2 pints low-fat yoghurt
3 tablespoons sugar
1 teaspoon lemon juice
2 slices pumpernickel bread
2 tablespoons honey
1 cup mandarin orange sections

Strain yoghurt and refrigerate for 4 hours. Stir in lemon

juice and sugar. Refrigerate for another 4 hours. Preheat oven to 375 degrees. Toast bread, crumble, and add honey. Press into bottom of 8 cups to make crust. Cover with yoghurt mixture. Add a couple of orange sections on top.

Chocolate Kisses

20 calories per serving
Makes 30 servings

3 tablespoons cocoa powder
½ cup confectioners' sugar
4 egg whites
½ teaspoon lemon juice
½ cup granulated sugar

Preheat oven to 250 degrees. Line a baking pan with waxed paper. Sift together cocoa powder and confectioners' sugar and set aside. Beat egg whites and lemon juice until soft peaks form. Add 1 ½ tablespoons granulated sugar and beat until stiff. Add remaining sugar and beat again until glossy. Fold in cocoa mixture. Spoon into small "kiss" shapes on baking sheet. Bake for 2 hours, then turn off oven and let set for 1 hour. Cool completely.

Blueberry Cake

125 calories per serving
Makes 15 servings

1 cup frozen blueberries, thawed
1 ½ tablespoons sugar
2 tablespoons margarine
2 tablespoons corn syrup
½ cup egg substitute
2 teaspoons almond extract
3 cups flour

1 ¼ teaspoons baking soda
1 ¼ cups nonfat sour cream
⅓ cup powdered sugar
2 teaspoons skimmed milk

Preheat oven to 375 degrees. Spray a fluted baking tin with nonfat cooking spray. Blend blueberries and sugar until smooth, set aside. In a medium bowl, combine margarine, corn syrup, egg substitute, and 1 teaspoon almond extract. Add flour, baking soda, and sour cream. Combine ¾ cup batter with blueberry mixture. Spread ⅔ of batter into pan, top with blueberry mix. Finish with remaining batter. Bake 40 minutes. Combine powdered sugar, 1 teaspoon almond extract, and skimmed milk. Drizzle over cooled cake.

Skimmed Milk Custard

90 calories per serving
Makes 4 servings

2 cups cold skimmed milk
1 tablespoon unflavoured gelatin
3 tablespoons sugar
1 teaspoon almond extract

Pour milk into saucepan and sprinkle gelatin in. Let stand for 5 minutes. Stir over low heat until gelatin is dissolved. Stir in sugar and cook for 3 minutes, stirring constantly. Remove from heat and stir in extract. Pour into 4 ramekins and chill until set.

S'mores Fudge

25 calories per serving
Makes 60 servings

8-ounce package reduced-fat chocolate baking chips

⅔ cup nonfat sweetened condensed milk
1 teaspoon vanilla extract
1 ⅓ cups miniature marshmallows
2 low-fat graham crackers, broken in small pieces

Line 8-inch baking pan with waxed paper. In nonstick saucepan, over low heat, stir chocolate chips and condensed milk until melted. Remove from heat and cool for 2 minutes, then stir in vanilla extract and 1 cup marshmallows. Pour into pan, sticking graham cracker pieces and remaining marshmallows into fudge. Refrigerate until firm. Peel off waxed paper, invert, and cut into 1-inch squares.

Sugar and Spice Doughnuts

125 calories per serving
Makes 10 servings

2 cups reduced-fat biscuit mix
3 tablespoons sugar
¼ teaspoon nutmeg
½ cup buttermilk
¼ cup egg substitute
1 tablespoon melted butter
¼ teaspoon cinnamon

Preheat oven to 425 degrees. Combine biscuit mix, 1 tablespoon sugar, nutmeg, buttermilk, and egg substitute. Knead dough on floured surface for 10 strokes. Roll out to ½-inch thickness. Cut with doughnut cutter and bake for 10 minutes. Combine remaining sugar and cinnamon. Brush doughnuts with butter and dip into cinnamon/sugar mixture.

Fruit Skewers with Mango Purée

80 calories per serving
Makes 4 servings

1 ripe mango, peeled, pitted, and chopped
1 tablespoon lime juice
½ pineapple, cored
1 papaya, peeled and seeded
2 kiwi, peeled and quartered

Place mango and lime juice in a food processor and blend. Cut pineapple and papaya into bite-sized chunks and thread on skewer with kiwi. To serve, spoon a little mango purée on four plates. Place cooked skewer on top.

Molasses Cookies

50 calories per serving
Makes 40 cookies

½ cup light molasses
⅓ cup shortening
2 cups flour
¼ cup brown sugar
1 tablespoon skim milk
1 teaspoon ginger
½ teaspoon baking powder

In a pan, heat molasses to boiling and stir in shortening until melted. Remove from heat and stir in flour, brown sugar, milk, ginger, and baking powder. Stir until mixture pulls away from pan. After dough cools, form into 1-inch thick log. Refrigerate until firm. Preheat oven to 350 degrees. Slice into ¼-inch slices. Bake on nonstick baking sheet for 10 minutes.

Index of Recipes